God's Rx

CHOICES: MANAGING CHRONIC PAIN

by

Jonnie Wright

Includes Leader's Guide

Copyright © 2008 by Jonnie Wright
Title & content by Jonnie Wright
jonnie@jonniewright.com
www.jonniewright.com
Cover design by Laura Taylor
ISBN: 978-0-9768950-1-5

All rights reserved. No part of this book may be reproduced or transmitted in any form or by any means, electronic or mechanical, including photocopying, recording, or any information storage and retrieval system without written permission from Jonnie Wright. www.jonniewright.com

All Scripture quotations, unless otherwise indicated, are taken from *NEW INTERNATIONAL VERSION.* Copyright © 1998 by Zondervan Reference Software developed from *The Holy Bible, New International Version,* Copyright © 1973, 1978, 1984 by The International Bible Society. (http://www.zondervan.com)

Printed in the United States of America

Books by Jonnie Wright

Lord, What do I do with Sammy?
(Christian teachers' workbook for difficult students)

God's Rx for Chronic Pain Series:
Book One: *The Silver Bullet*
Book Two: *Choices*

TABLE OF CONTENTS

INTRODUCTION... 5

CHAPTER ONE.. 7
Victimized by Circumstances or Rejuvenated by Faith

CHAPTER TWO... 29
Make a Loud Noise or Sing a New Song

CHAPTER THREE.. 51
Curse Your Enemies or Bless Your God

CHAPTER FOUR.. 73
Worldly Cares or Heavenly Promises

LEADER'S GUIDE.. 95
Memorizing Scripture

GOD'S Rx FOR CHRONIC PAIN SERIES........... 104

ACKNOWLEDGEMENTS

No one can write in a vacuum, and I surely could not have completed this book without the loving encouragement and assistance from the following people:

Wilma (Winnie) Clark who taught me how to write as she edited this book; Laura Taylor who took picture after picture until the book cover became a masterpiece; and Janice Haller who completed last minute Scripture research.

Along with these three individuals, I want to acknowledge the many friends who encouraged and supported me so willingly: Jeanette Bush, David Cartt, Leslie Davison Barbie Eslin, Deborah Geyer, Marilyn Ginter, Christi Howarth, Michael Loden, Irene Sharpnack, Shari Whitaker, and Lori and Kevin Wilhelm. Thanks to you all!

INTRODUCTION

Change is as inevitable as death and taxes. Our choices reflect the inescapability of what change asks of us. Chronic illness threatens our life-style, adds to our financial burdens, stresses our relationships, and interrupts our life. Often our choices alter our physical and emotional state so much that, in time, we become strangers to our former selves. Yet, we must live as victors not victims.

Thankfully, the Bible is more than just a first aid book for spiritual boo-boos. Through Scripture, we learn of the promised, unfathomable riches of God's love, mercy and justice. We are inspired by the stories of men and women who failed as often as they succeeded, but whose faithfulness was rewarded. Because the Bible is the inerrant word of God, Scripture can help us through our struggles and difficult choices. But, do we allot enough time in Scripture study to realign our perspective with God's will?

The good news is that we do not need to be Biblical scholars to discover the truths found in Scripture. *Choices: Managing Chronic Pain* offers short studies, minimum writing, and maximum application. The simplicity of the *Choices* format encourages we who are in chronic pain to consider **whatever is true, whatever is noble, whatever is right, whatever is pure, whatever is lovely, whatever is admirable--if anything is excellent or praiseworthy—** [to] **think about such things.** (Phil. 4:8)

How to use this book:
Each one-page study provides Scripture verse(s) taken from the New International Version (NIV) of the Bible. Questions challenge you to apply Biblical principles to your past, present, and future actions. Each chapter emphasizes a Biblical character whose life choices determined who he was, how his life changed because of

his choices, and what relevance his choices have for us today. A journal topic with Scripture reference is found at the end of each one-page study for further insight.

A case for journaling:
Everywhere we turn we are encouraged to journal. From the food we eat, the health symptoms we endure, the exercise routine we schedule, even the number of daily steps we take, all require a record on paper of our thoughts and feelings. Effective journaling helps us stop and look at what we're doing, how we're feeling, and who we are at that moment. Whether we write two words or two pages, journaling encourages us to consider our challenges, our responses, our victories, and our self-promises. Journaling inspires us to record God's mini-miracles, His rescues, and His involvement in our life. Journaling records the today we may not remember tomorrow.

In order to receive the greatest benefit from this study, you must have a relationship with God through Jesus Christ. If Jesus is not Lord of your life, invite Him into your heart today to assure your Salvation and claim future intimacy with Him.

A prayer for Salvation:
Father God, I know you love me and have a plan for my life. I acknowledge that I am a sinner and that I cannot solve my life's problems. I recognize that Jesus Christ died for my sins, and by doing so provided me with eternal life. Please Jesus, come into my heart and life, make me whole, and help me live in the truth of your saving grace. Thank you Jesus, that you've come into my life right now, you've forgiven my sins, and that you will be with me through all of my life's challenges. Amen.

* Throughout this book, the terms "Israelites," "Hebrews," and "Jews" will refer to the nation of God's chosen people established through the descendants of Jacob, whom God renamed Israel.

CHAPTER ONE

Victimized by Circumstances or Rejuvenated by Faith

Joseph's story relates the best of times and the worst of times. He was his father's favorite son. This partiality made his eleven brothers angry and resentful. Thus, when chance came, they sold him to slavers headed for Egypt.

Once in Egypt, Joseph was sold as a slave to a very rich man. He rose to a position second only to his master. Alas, his handsomeness attracted his master's wife and she attempted to seduce him. When rebuked, she declared rape, and Joseph was thrown into Pharaoh's prison.

As a prisoner, Joseph rose to foreman in charge of all the other prisoners. He interpreted the Pharaoh's butcher and wine taster's dreams correctly, and two years later he was summoned to the palace to interpret Pharaoh's dream. Upon the fulfillment of his interpretation, Joseph rose from jailbird to ruler of Egypt, second only to Pharaoh himself.

Joseph certainly was beset by cruel circumstances as his status was stolen from him again and again. He refused, however, to be a victim, but honored God no matter what the situation. Throughout his many struggles, Joseph knew God was working in his life, so he continued to worship God and follow His laws. As ruler of Egypt, Joseph forgave his brothers with these words: **You intended to harm me, but God intended it for good to accomplish what is now being done...** (Gen. 50:20a) We find no victimization in the life of Joseph, only his rejuvenation of faith in God. We too can rise above our circumstances when we choose to have faith and take action through God's promises.

Joseph: Man of Circumstance #1

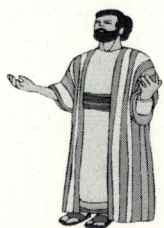

³**Now Israel loved Joseph more than any of his other sons, because he had been born to him in his old age; and he made a richly ornamented robe for him. ⁴When his brothers saw that their father loved him more than any of them, they hated him and could not speak a kind word to him.** (Gen. 37:3-4)

Jealousy and favoritism pervert normal family relationships. Joseph fed his brothers' resentment by sharing two dreams that portrayed his ruling over them. (Gen. 37:5-11)

☦ Do you envy or resent a family member or a friend? Pray for them right now. If no resentments, why not?

☦ Joseph's dreams were prophetic and sustained him in his many trials. But most people's dreams are symbolic. Consider your dreams. What do they tell you?

☦ How does God most frequently communicate with you: dreams, prayer, Scriptures, sermons, friends, family, group interaction, or circumstances? Explain.

JOURNAL: LUKE 15:25-32 HOW DO YOU RESPOND TO JEALOUSY, YOURS OR SOMEONE ELSE'S?

Rejuvenated by Faith #1

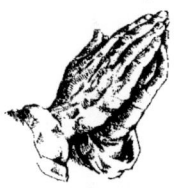

²³Love the LORD, all his saints! The LORD preserves the faithful, but the proud he pays back in full. ²⁴Be strong and take heart, all you who hope in the LORD. (Ps. 31:23-24)

✞ Why are you called a "saint" when you don't do everything perfectly?

✞ If you can't be perfect, how can you be faithful?

✞ When you are weakened by your illness and demoralized by your circumstances, how can you "take heart"?

✞ Ps. 31:5 states, *Into your hands I commit my spirit; redeem me, O LORD, the God of truth.* Where can you apply the truth of this Scripture in your life: during a health crisis, struggling with financial issues, feeling alone in your pain, dealing with family circumstances, being overwhelmed by your situation, adjusting to your changing life-style?

JOURNAL: PS. 27 WHEN ARE YOU AFRAID? HOW DO YOU DEAL WITH YOUR FEARS? HOW CAN GOD HELP?

Joseph: Man of Circumstance #2

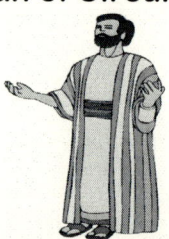

²⁶Judah said to his brothers, "What will we gain if we kill our brother and cover up his blood? ²⁷Come, let's sell him to the Ishmaelites and not lay our hands on him; after all, he is our brother, our own flesh and blood." His brothers agreed. (Gen. 37:26-27)

✞ Joseph's brothers chose to sell him instead of killing him. Was this due to their morality or God's plan? Explain.

✞ When have you experienced betrayal or rejection by someone you loved? Have you ever done any rejecting?

✞ Everyone lies at some point in his or her life. When have you lied to keep yourself out of trouble? How did you feel?

✞ When you discover someone's deceit, what actions have you, or can you, take? Are these strategies effective? Explain.

JOURNAL: PHIL. 4:6-9 WHAT MAKES YOU ANXIOUS? WHAT DOES SCRIPTURE SUGGEST YOU DO?

Rejuvenated by Faith #2

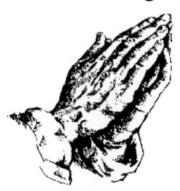

For the LORD loves the just and will not forsake his faithful ones. They will be protected forever, but the offspring of the wicked will be cut off; (Ps. 37:28)

✞ What has God promised to you, oh faithful one?

✞ In Psalm 37, the wicked being "cut off" is declared five times. What justice will the wicked receive? Can you determine who is wicked and who is not? Explain.

✞ Give an example where good things happened to a "bad" person.

✞ Give an example where bad things happened to a good person. Why does God allow this?

✞ What spectacular physical healing have you personally seen happen to someone else? If never, why not?

JOURNAL: PHIL. 2:1-11 WITH WHAT ATTITUDE DOES GOD WANT YOU TO LIVE? HOW CAN YOU ACCOMPLISH THIS?

Joseph: Man of Circumstance #3

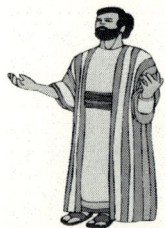

Now Joseph had been taken down to Egypt. Potiphar, an Egyptian who was one of Pharaoh's officials, the captain of the guard, bought him from the Ishmaelites who had taken him there. (Gen. 39:1)

Potiphar, a shrewd man, recognized Joseph as a man of God. He entrusted his entire household and all that he owned to Joseph's care. Joseph graduated from slave to administrator.

☦ How could Potiphar know Joseph was a man of God?

☦ Do those around you know that you are a man/woman of God? How? If not, why not?

☦ When you meet new people, are they aware of your illness? How? If not, then how do you share the knowledge of your daily struggles with them?

☦ Does your attitude or behavior draw attention to your illness? Does your life-style? How? Should it?

JOURNAL: ROM. 10:8-13 WHAT DOES IT MEAN TO BELIEVE?

Rejuvenated by Faith #3

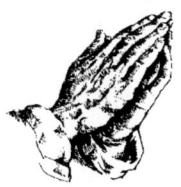

He will cover you with his feathers, and under his wings you will find refuge; his faithfulness will be your shield and rampart. (Ps. 91:4)

☦ Picture baby birds nestling under the safety of their mother's wings. When does God's protection feel like that of a mother bird?

☦ With twenty-five sightings of "eagle" in the Bible (NIV), this bird's qualities consider contemplation. Which eagle attributes would you desire: swooping down, stirring the nest, hovering, soaring, or riding the air currents? Why?

☦ From what would you have God shield you? Explain?

☦ What visual picture of God do you like best: a nesting hen, a soaring eagle, a protective shield, a well-built fort, a healthy immune system, or an impenetrable force field? Why?

JOURNAL: PS. 42:1-11 WHEN HAVE YOU BEEN ABLE TO DEFEAT DEPRESSION? HOW? IF NOT, HOW DOES DEPRESSION DEFEAT YOU? WHAT CAN YOU DO?

Joseph: Man of Circumstance #4

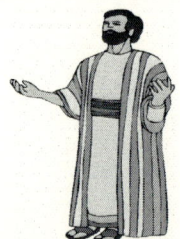

⁶...Now Joseph was well-built and handsome, ⁷and after a while his master's wife took notice of Joseph and said, "Come to bed with me!" (Gen. 39:6b,7)

A young man being propositioned by a woman of power seems like an enviable position. Joseph, however, recognized this temptation for what it was—sin against God. He chose to flee rather than be flattered.

✞ How do you respond to flattery?

✞ 1 Cor. 10:13 says, *No temptation has seized you except what is common to man. And God is faithful; he will not let you be tempted beyond what you can bear. But when you are tempted, he will also provide a way out so that you can stand up under it.* What temptations do you struggle with?

✞ What does 1 Cor. 10:13 promise will happen when you are tempted? Why would God provide an escape from temptation?

JOURNAL: PS. 65 HOW DOES GOD PROVIDE FOR YOU ACCORDING TO THIS PSALM?

Rejuvenated by Faith #4

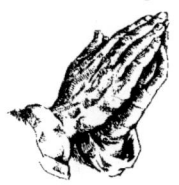

³Let love and faithfulness never leave you; bind them around your neck, write them on the tablet of your heart. ⁴Then you will win favor and a good name in the sight of God and man. (Prov. 3:3-4)

✞ Who is the source of your love, and of your faithfulness? Who can write these qualities on your heart?

✞ Where do you find the strength necessary to love the unlikable, the ugly, and the unacceptable? Do you see yourself in one of these three categories? Explain.

✞ What behavior will win you favor with man? Can you produce the behavior necessary to sustain this esteem? If yes, how? If no, explain why not.

✞ How do you win favor with God? Will it be your conduct or your heart that is most important to Him?

✞ Why does God love you?

JOURNAL: LUKE 5:27-32 WHAT SIZE IS YOUR COMMITMENT?

Joseph: Man of Circumstance #5

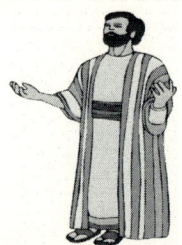

¹⁹When his master heard the story his wife told him, saying, "This is how your slave treated me," he burned with anger. ²⁰Joseph's master took him and put him in prison, the place where the king's prisoners were confined. (Gen. 39:19-20)

Once more Joseph's liberty was snatched away as he found himself in Pharaoh's prison. And it's Joseph's faithfulness to God's laws that again elevated his status as the head guard promoted him to manager of the entire prison.

✞ What was Joseph's most important resource: good luck, good looks, administration skills, faith, obedience, or God's favor? Explain.

✞ What is your most important resource? Why?

✞ Explain Rom. 8:28 in terms of your illness, *And we know that in all things God works for the good of those who love him, who have been called according to his purpose.*

JOURNAL: PS. 3 WHEN DO YOU FEEL GOD'S ASSURANCE? WHEN IS IT AVAILABLE TO YOU?

Rejuvenated by Faith #5

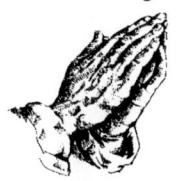

His master replied, "Well done, good and faithful servant! You have been faithful with a few things; I will put you in charge of many things. Come and share your master's happiness!" (Matt. 25:23)

This Scripture is taken from the parable of the talents in which a traveling merchant entrusts five talents (a unit of money) to one servant, two to another, and one to the last. The merchant returns home and each servant reports on how he invested the money. Those who made a profit received praise those who do not received judgment. (Matt. 25:14-30)

☦ What have you done with the aptitudes, abilities, and skills God has given you? How have you "made a profit" in God's name?

☦ How does your illness affect your capability to use these gifts God has given you?

☦ In what behavior can you say you're reasonably faithful? How do you stay committed? If not, why not?

JOURNAL: JOHN 10:1-16 DOES JESUS CARE ABOUT YOU? HOW DO YOU KNOW? WHAT EXPERIENCES HAVE YOU HAD THAT SHOW HIS CARE?

Joseph: Man of Circumstance #6

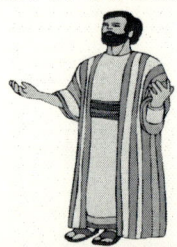

7So he [Joseph] asked Pharaoh's officials who were in custody with him in his master's house, "Why are your faces so sad today?" 8"We both had dreams," they answered, "but there is no one to interpret them." Then Joseph said to them, "Do not interpretations belong to God? Tell me your dreams." (Gen. 40:7-8)

Dreams are 95% symbolic, 5% prophetic. God gave Joseph an amazing gift to predict the future by interpreting dreams. God can use your dreams as well, but remember that most dreams will be metaphoric rather than prophetic no matter how real they seem.

- ✞ Share a memorable or distressing dream. If you have trouble remembering dreams, write them down before you get out of bed in the morning.

- ✞ There are many books on dreams. Most of them do not have a godly foundation. As Joseph pointed out, only God can interpret dreams. Can you discover the meaning of your dreams? How? Is it important to you to understand their meaning? Explain.

JOURNAL: PS. 8 MEDITATE ON HOW MAJESTIC IS YOUR GOD. ADD WORDS OF PRAISE TO THIS PSALM.

Rejuvenated by Faith #6

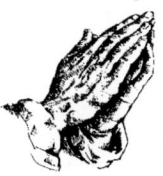

[11]Never be lacking in zeal, but keep your spiritual fervor, serving the Lord. [12]Be joyful in hope, patient in affliction, faithful in prayer. (Rom. 12:11-12)

- ☦ When do you feel zealous for the Lord? If not, why not?

- ☦ How can you keep your "spiritual fervor" when you're in pain? What attitude do you desire?

- ☦ When do you find yourself hopeful? If never, why not?

- ☦ How can you be "patient" in your chronic pain state?

- ☦ Which statement do you agree with? I pray for a specific length of time every day. I pray when the need arises. I pray for my meals. I pray for others' specific needs. I pray at church services & Bible studies. I forget to pray. How do you feel about your commitment to prayer?

JOURNAL: PS. 143 WHAT DOES GOD'S WORD SAY ABOUT AFFLICTION? ARE YOU COMFORTED? EXPLAIN.

Joseph: Man of Circumstance #7

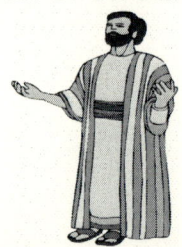

Pharaoh sent for Joseph and said, *¹⁵"...I had a dream, and no one can interpret it. But I have heard it said of you that when you hear a dream you can interpret it." ¹⁶"I cannot do it," Joseph replied to Pharaoh, "but God will give Pharaoh the answer he desires."* (Gen. 41:15b, 16)

Joseph's circumstances brought him into the presence of Pharaoh, where Joseph did not boast but reminded everyone in Pharaoh's court that only God can interpret dreams.

✞ How would you feel if you stood before the President of the U.S. and he asked for your opinion?

✞ Joseph took no credit for his gift. When have you given God the credit for a talent or ability you've used lately?

✞ Do your medications influence the content or number of your dreams? If your dreams are frightening, how can knowing God speaks to you through them (Joel 2:28) comfort you? If you find no comfort, why not?

JOURNAL: PS. 19 HOW DOES CREATION PROVE GOD'S EXISTENCE? HOW DO YOUR DREAMS?

Rejuvenated by Faith #7

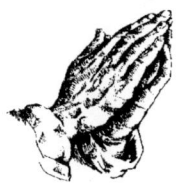

God, who has called you into fellowship with his Son Jesus Christ our Lord, is faithful. (1 Cor. 1:9)

✞ Why is it important to you that God is faithful?

✞ Where do you see His faithfulness in your life?

✞ When is God's faithfulness revealed in your illness?

✞ When are you faithful to God in your finances?

✞ Which relationships depend on your authenticity and truth? Which ones don't? Why?

✞ How does your illness hamper your believability as a Christian to other people? If it does not, why not?

JOURNAL: LUKE 9:1-10 HOW AND WHEN DO YOU MINISTER TO OTHERS? HOW DOES HELPING OTHERS HELP YOU? WHEN DOES IT NOT?

Joseph: Man of Circumstance #8

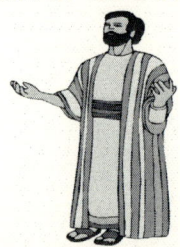

[39] Then Pharaoh said to Joseph, "Since God has made all this known to you, there is no one so discerning and wise as you. [40] You shall be in charge of my palace, and all my people are to submit to your orders. Only with respect to the throne will I be greater than you." (Gen. 41:39-40)

Joseph's rise to power was not achieved by his own efforts. God had a plan. He wanted His people to survive the famine and learn the lessons of Egypt.

✟ How do you explain Joseph's success? He was lucky. He knew what to say. He was likable. He prayed a lot. He was crafted by God to fulfill a great purpose? Explain.

✟ For what purpose have you been crafted? How do you know? If you do not know, how can you find out?

✟ Does your health help or hinder this God's purpose? How?

JOURNAL: MATT. 6:19-34 WHAT ARE YOUR SPIRITUAL PRIORITIES? DO THEY ALIGN WITH GOD'S WILL?

Rejuvenated by Faith #8

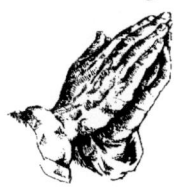

¹²Dear friends, do not be surprised at the painful trial you are suffering, as though something strange were happening to you. ¹³ But rejoice that you participate in the sufferings of Christ, so that you may be overjoyed when his glory is revealed. (1 Peter 4:12-13)

Peter's words remind us that we will suffer. He suggests appropriate action, *So then, those who suffer according to God's will should commit themselves to their faithful Creator and continue to do good.* (1 Peter 4:19)

☦ What does "doing good" look like to you?

☦ How can you "do good" when you are suffering?

☦ Is your suffering: punishment, discipline, dumb luck, inferior body parts, a test, a task, Satan's trick, or God's plan? How does your answer make you feel?

☦ What does your rejoicing look like when you are in pain?

JOURNAL: JOHN 13:3-17 WHEN ARE YOU WILLING TO SERVE OTHERS? HOW DOES THAT MAKE YOU FEEL?

Joseph: Man of Circumstance #9

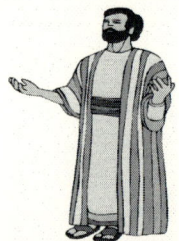

³Then ten of Joseph's brothers went down to buy grain from Egypt. ⁸Although Joseph recognized his brothers, they did not recognize him. (Gen. 42:3, 8)

The worldwide famine reached Canaan. Egypt was the only country with food, so Jacob sent ten of his eleven sons to purchase food. Benjamin, the youngest, stayed home.

☦ Why would Joseph pretend not to know his brothers? He was surprised seeing them. He wanted to toy with them. He wanted to punish them. He was unsure how he felt.

☦ Have you ever come face-to-face with your abuser? How did you feel? If you have never been abused, how could you comfort someone who has?

☦ When do you pretend to be well? Why do you feel you must? Would appearing sick give you any advantages? Explain.

JOURNAL: 1 PETER 1:3-9 OF WHAT WORTH ARE THE TRIALS YOU SUFFER? OF WHAT REWARDS ARE YOU GUARANTEED?

Rejuvenated by Faith #9

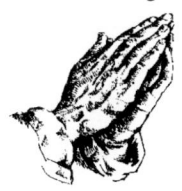

Do not be afraid of what you are about to suffer. I tell you, the devil will put some of you in prison to test you, and you will suffer persecution for ten days. Be faithful, even to the point of death, and I will give you the crown of life. (Rev. 2:10)

✞ Does your illness cause you fear? How? If not, why not? Does God waste your suffering? Explain.

✞ Do you suffer persecution because of your illness? Because you are a Christian? Explain.

✞ Can you overcome every obstacle your illness generates? How? If you cannot, what do you need to know or to do?

✞ Have you found a spiritual reason for your physical illness? If so, what is it? If you do not know, ask yourself why God would allow you to be sick, remembering that He is Spirit and you are flesh.

JOURNAL: ISA. 40:1-11 HOW DO THESE WORDS COMFORT YOU? IF THEY DO NOT, WHY NOT? WHAT ELSE DO YOU NEED?

Joseph: Man of Circumstance #10

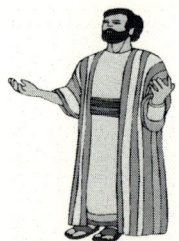

"So then, it was not you who sent me here, but God. He made me father to Pharaoh, lord of his entire household and ruler of all Egypt." (Gen. 45:8)

After various ploys, Joseph finally revealed himself to his brothers. He recognized his brothers' repentance by their behavior. Their choice to sell him had caused them years of personal grief. Joseph's forgiveness freed them from the crippling guilt they had lived with for so many years.

☦ What poor decisions in your past have crippled you in your present circumstances? Are you able to repair any of the damage? What would you have done differently?

☦ How do you recognize repentance: a changed attitude, a changed behavior, an apology given, a "sorry" spoken? When do you know repentance is sincere?

☦ How do you deal with guilt? Has your illness ever caused you to feel guilty? How? If not, how do you avoid feeling guilty about your chronic illness?

JOURNAL: PS. 51 GOD DOES NOT WANT YOU TO BE BURDENED WITH GUILT? WHY?

Rejuvenated by Faith #10

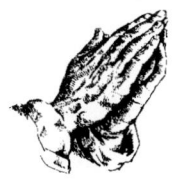

This calls for patient endurance on the part of the saints who obey God's commandments and remain faithful to Jesus. (Rev. 14:12)

✞ What does "patient endurance" mean to you?

✞ When are you patient? What is patience's reward? What happens if you're not patient? How do you feel then?

✞ What attitudes or behaviors would you expect from a "saint," (remember only Jesus is perfect)?

✞ How do you remain faithful to Jesus: tithe, go to church, stay cheerful, read the Bible, pray for people, pray for healing, belong to a Bible study, do good works, worship God on Sundays, help someone needy?

✞ What would you like to be doing when God calls you home?

JOURNAL: LUKE 24:13-32 WHAT WOULD AN AFTERNOON WITH JESUS BE LIKE?

CHAPTER TWO

Make a Loud Noise or Sing a New Song

God called Moses to a momentous task. Free the Israelites from the bondage of Egypt. Lead over a million ex-slaves to the Promised Land. Establish a new system of government. Teach the people how to worship holy God.

To be prepared with the necessary skills and abilities, Moses would be raised as an Egyptian, kill an Egyptian, and flee for his life to the desert. For forty years God would hone Moses' skills as a shepherd in the desert. Not until he was eighty would Moses encounter God in the burning bush.

As God laid out His plans for the deliverance of the Hebrew nation, Moses' response to God was not "How great thou are," but "Send someone else!" God, however, did not give up on Moses, but walked him step by step into a trusting relationship through the experiences of a resistant Hebrew nation, a mocking Egyptian Pharaoh, a flight into the desert with over a million people, and a trap at the edge of the Red Sea. With their backs against the sea and the Egyptians hard on their trail, Moses changed his tune from, "I can't" to "God will deliver us!"

Moses quaked before the task God called him to; yet from his loud noise came a new song. His own weaknesses blinded him to the strengths of God. And how like Moses we are. We worry about our own shortcomings instead of trusting in our God's ability to see His works accomplished through us.

Moses: Man of Noise #1

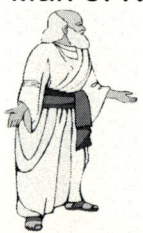

But Moses said to God, "Who am I, that I should go to Pharaoh and bring the Israelites out of Egypt?" (Ex. 3:11)

God revealed Himself to Moses in an unconsumed burning bush. God spoke to Moses explaining His plan for the deliverance of the Israelite nation from Egyptian slavery. And what was Moses' response? Whining! He could not see himself being a part of God's plan. He forgot to look at the size of his God.

☦ Has God revealed His plan for your life? If not, are you: waiting quietly to hear His direction? Saying yes to every church activity? Burning out in what you thought was God's work? Or doing your own thing while waiting for God to bless your efforts?

☦ Moses put God in a box the size of his own anticipation. How have you boxed God into the size of your pain?

☦ When have you whined to God? Why?

JOURNAL: PS. 46 WHEN DO YOU FEEL FEAR? WHERE CAN YOUR SOUL FIND REST FROM THIS DISQUIET?

Sing A New Song #1

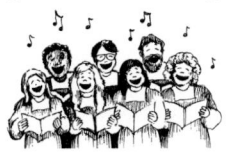

³Sing to him a new song; play skillfully, and shout for joy. ⁴For the word of the LORD is right and true; he is faithful in all he does. (Ps. 33:3-4)

✟ This Scripture lists 3 ways to worship God: sing, play, and shout. Which action fits your style of worship?

✟ God models faithfulness in His work of Salvation through Jesus Christ. In what areas of your life have you seen God's faithfulness?

✟ How does knowing that God is faithful encourage you when those "bad" days occur?

✟ Has God ever been unfaithful to you? Have you ever been unfaithful to Him?

✟ How do you know God is not punishing you with your illness? Read Isa. 53:4-5. Who do these words refer to?

JOURNAL: JOHN 20:1-18 WHEN HAVE YOU FELT DESPAIR? WHAT DID YOU DO? HOW DID YOUR JOY RETURN? WHY DID IT?

Moses: Man of Noise #2

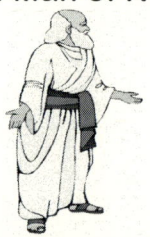

Moses said to God, "Suppose I go to the Israelites and say to them, 'The God of your fathers has sent me to you,' and they ask me, 'What is his name?' Then what shall I tell them?" (Ex. 3:13)

God's reply to Moses' questions was, *I AM WHO I AM. This is what you are to say to the Israelites: "I AM has sent me to you."* (Ex. 3:14) But Moses still doubted that God could pull off a rescue operation using him.

✟ In ancient times, a person's name held great importance. How is God's name, *I AM WHO I AM*, significant to you?

✟ The Israelites were slaves for 400 years before God freed them. During those years, many prayers seemed to go unanswered. Do you have any unanswered prayers? How patient are you in waiting for answers?

✟ When has your life taken a new direction in response to an unexpected circumstance? What was your reaction?

JOURNAL: 2 CHRON. 20:15-24 HOW DOES KNOWING THAT GOD WILL FIGHT YOUR BATTLES HELP YOU IN TIMES OF DISTRESS?

Sing A New Song #2

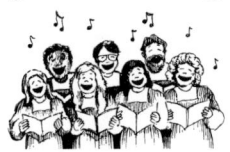

²*He lifted me out of the slimy pit, out of the mud and mire; he set my feet on a rock and gave me a firm place to stand. ³He put a new song in my mouth, a hymn of praise to our God. Many will see and fear and put their trust in the LORD.* (Ps. 40:2-3)

✞ In what slimy pit do you find yourself? Are you knee-deep, up to your armpits, in over your head? Explain.

✞ Jesus is your firm rock on which to stand. How does knowing this truth put a new song in your heart?

✞ What comes out of your mouth? Does God hear you complaining and whining or praise and thanking?

✞ Which helps you more in your present circumstances: remembering God's faithfulness in the past or claiming God's promises for the future? Explain.

✞ When do doubts rob you of joy in the Lord? Explain.

JOURNAL: JOHN 20:24-29 WHEN DO YOU HAVE DOUBTS?

Moses: Man of Noise #3

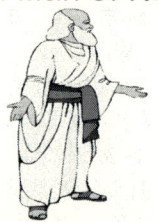

Moses answered, "What if they do not believe me or listen to me and say, 'The LORD did not appear to you'?" (Ex. 4:1)

In Exodus 3, God gave Moses His vision, His motivation, His plan. Yet again Moses questioned God. God responded by turning Moses' staff into a snake and back into a staff again. He made Moses' hand leprous then healed it.

☦ Is Moses' question reasonable, or is he: worrying about other people's approval, thinking of past rejections, lacking trust in God, or feeling inadequate? Explain.

☦ How would you have reacted to these two miracles God performed for Moses?

☦ Notice how God is outlining the job He's asking Moses to do. Remember God never changes. How does He take care of the events and details in your life, or are you in such a muddle you cannot tell?

JOURNAL: PS. 34 HOW IS YOUR SPIRIT AFFIRMED WHILE READING THIS PSALM? IF IT IS NOT, WHO ELSE IS THERE TO AFFIRM YOU?

Sing A New Song #3

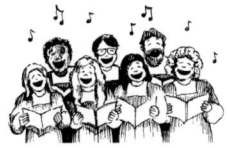

¹Sing to the LORD a new song; sing to the LORD, all the earth. ²Sing to the LORD, praise his name; proclaim his salvation day after day. (Ps. 96:1-2)

Do you have a favorite song, maybe one you sing in the shower? What do you like about this song: the beat, the words, the instruments, the blend of voices? Ever wonder what God likes to hear? God created music. He gave birds a song to sing, crickets a noise to chirp, cows a desire to moo. How much more pleased He must be to hear our songs of adoration and praise.

☦ What is your favorite worship song? Hum it to yourself now.

☦ What character qualities of God, such as salvation or compassion, are expressed in this song?

☦ What phrases tug at your heart and bring you closer to your Holy Father God?

JOURNAL: A HEBREW ACROSTIC STARTS EACH LINE WITH THE BEGINNING OF THE NEXT ALPHABET LETTER. WRITE YOUR OWN PSALM USING THE LETTERS FROM *FAITH*, *WISDOM*, OR *GRACE*.

Moses: Man of Noise # 4

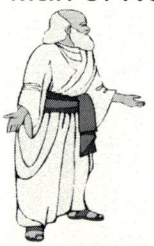

But Moses said, "O Lord, please send someone else to do it." (Ex. 4:13)

God spoke from a burning bush, gave Moses His most holy Name, turned Moses' staff to a snake, made his hand leprous, reminded Moses that He had made his mouth, and outlined His plan from start to finish. Moses' response was pitiful. Though angry, God sent Aaron to speak for Moses.

☦ Have you ever been asked to do something you were sure you couldn't do? How did you respond?

☦ What do you think is behind all of Moses' excuses: his speech impairment, his insecurity, his stubbornness, his humility, his pride? Explain.

☦ When you decline to participate in a new, unfamiliar situation, do you offer excuses or rational explanations? How do you feel after you say no, or do you say yes even though you know you'll probably be miserable?

JOURNAL: LUKE 7:1-10 DOUBT IS NOT THE OPPOSITE OF FAITH, IT IS ONE OF ITS BUILDING BLOCKS. DO YOU AGREE? EXPLAIN.

Sing A New Song #4

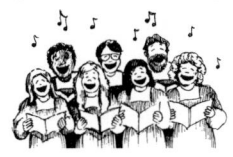

¹Sing to the LORD a new song, for he has done marvelous things; his right hand and his holy arm have worked salvation for him. ²The LORD has made his salvation known and revealed his righteousness to the nations. (Ps. 98:1-2)

☦ What marvelous things has God done in your life? How have your attitudes and behaviors changed as a result of these grand things God has done?

☦ God reveals the salvation and righteousness of Jesus Christ to the nations. How does God make known His presence to you?

☦ What difference has God's revelation of Jesus Christ made in how you deal with pain? If none, why not?

☦ Consider the statement, "God is His own evangelist." Can this be true? How? If you disagree, why?

JOURNAL: JOHN 12:12-18 WHAT EXPERIENCES ASSURE YOU THAT JESUS IS YOUR LORD? IF NONE, HOW CAN YOU BE CONFIDENT OF YOUR SALVATION?

Moses: Man of Noise #5

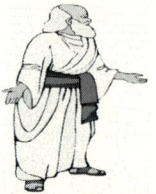

²²Moses returned to the LORD and said, "O Lord, why have you brought trouble upon this people? Is this why you sent me? ²³Ever since I went to Pharaoh to speak in your name, he has brought trouble upon this people, and you have not rescued your people at all." (Ex. 5:22-23)

Moses finally obeyed and declared God's message to Pharaoh. Pharaoh retaliated by demanding the Hebrew slaves find their own straw to make bricks. Moses expressed an I-told-you-so attitude to God.

✞ How do you feel when accused of doing something for which you are innocent: like a martyr, like a scapegoat, like running away, like running to God, like being defensive, or like getting angry? Explain.

✞ Pharaoh defied God's message and chose the consequences. In what ways do you resist the circumstances of your illness instead of walking with God in them?

✞ Does knowing God's big picture help with your daily decisions? Explain.

JOURNAL: PS. 34: WHAT ARE THE QUALITIES OF GOD THAT ENCOURAGE YOU? EXPLAIN WHY.

Sing A New Song #5

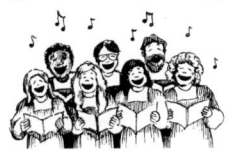

I will sing a new song to you, O God; on the ten-stringed lyre I will make music to you, (Ps. 144:9)

☦ Must a praise song have words to it or can the song be instruments only? Explain.

☦ What limitations does your illness place on your ability to praise? How do you overcome these snags?

☦ Make a list of ways you can praise God. Practice daily.

☦ Ps. 143:8 beseeches God to **Let the morning bring me word of your unfailing love, for I have put my trust in you. Show me the way I should go, for to you I lift up my soul.** How do you feel when you wake up in the morning? What do you tell yourself as you face the day?

☦ What Scripture can you cling to that will help you get out of bed?

JOURNAL: PS. 95: WE ARE THE SHEEP WHO FILL GOD'S PASTURE. WHAT DOES GOD PROVIDE FOR US?

Moses: Man of Noise #6

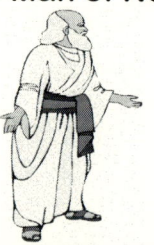

But Moses said to the LORD, "If the Israelites will not listen to me, why would Pharaoh listen to me, since I speak with faltering lips?" (Ex. 6:12)

Perplexed, Moses scowled at the cruel circumstances the Israelites faced. Increased brutality was the only change he saw. Pharaoh was not impressed, and the Israelites no longer believed the words of deliverance Moses spoke. Not seeing success, Moses again complained that God had made a big mistake in choosing him.

☦ What was Moses' biggest grievance: his own reputation, the Hebrew's suffering, Pharaoh's mocking, God's inactivity? Explain.

☦ Moses' complaint reflects a lack of confidence in whom: himself, Israelites, Pharaoh, God? Do you and Moses share this lack of confidence? Explain.

☦ What circumstances in your post interfere with who you want to be? Can God use you anyway? How?

JOURNAL: LUKE 15:11-24 WHY DOES THE FATHER FORGIVE HIS SON? WHY DOES GOD FORGIVE YOU?

Sing A New Song #6

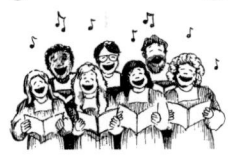

¹Praise the LORD. Sing to the LORD a new song, his praise in the assembly of the saints... ⁴For the LORD takes delight in his people; he crowns the humble with salvation. (Ps. 149: 1, 4)

✝ When you sing with other Christians, "the assembly of the saints," do you delight in your praise and worship? Does God? Why?

✝ If you cannot join other Christians singing at church, Christmas carols, or other events, what else can you do?

✝ Easton's Illustrated Dictionary concludes its definition of humility with the statement, it is a "...great paradox [contradiction] in Christianity that it makes humility the avenue to glory." Why does God crown the humble?

✝ Does being chronically ill make you humble or does it make you something else? Can you change? How?

JOURNAL: MATT. 14:22-33 WHEN HAS YOUR LIFE BEEN STORMY? HOW DID YOU SURVIVE? WHAT CAN YOU CHANGE BEFORE YOUR NEXT STORM HITS?

Moses: Man of Song #7

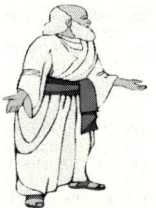

¹³Moses answered the people, "Do not be afraid. Stand firm and you will see the deliverance the LORD will bring you today. The Egyptians you see today you will never see again. ¹⁴The LORD will fight for you; you need only to be still." (Ex. 14:13-14)

Moses changed his tune. He witnessed the ten plagues God brought upon the Egyptians that culminated in freedom for the Hebrews. He viewed the pillar of cloud by day and the pillar of fire by night that separated the Egyptian army from the fleeing Hebrews. Finally, Moses believed that God could part the Red Sea for His people.

☦ When has God parted the Red Sea in your life?

☦ How has your faith grown since this "Red Sea" experience? I know myself better. I trust God more. I do not fear the next crisis. I trust God's people more. I live one day at a time. Explain.

☦ When you're in pain, how can you "only be still"?

JOURNAL: PS. 142 WHEN YOU FEEL OVERWHELMED, WHY DOES GOD LISTEN TO YOUR COMPLAINTS? DO YOU LISTEN FOR HIS ANSWERS?

Sing A New Song #7

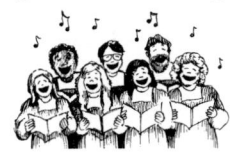

⁵Let the saints rejoice in this honor and sing for joy on their beds. ⁶May the praise of God be in their mouths and a double-edged sword in their hands. (Ps. 149:5-6)

✞ How can God delight in you when you're in confined in bed? Explain.

✞ Hebrews 4:12 compares a double-edged sword to the word of God: *For the word of God is living and active. Sharper than any double-edged sword, it penetrates even to dividing soul and spirit, joints and marrow; it judges the thoughts and attitudes of the heart.* When God judges your thoughts and attitudes about Him, what does He find?

✞ If you are in bed, how can you wield this double-edged sword, the word of God? Does it matter where you are?

✞ Psalms 145-150 are songs of praise to the Lord. Choose one and add your own words of praise.

JOURNAL: 1 KINGS 19:3-18 WHEN YOU FEEL LIKE GIVING UP, WHAT CAN GOD'S WORDS DO FOR YOU?

Moses: Man of Song #8

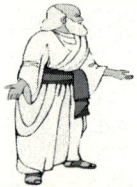

¹Then Moses and the Israelites sang this song to the LORD: "I will sing to the LORD, for he is highly exalted. The horse and its rider he has hurled into the sea. ²The LORD is my strength and my song; he has become my salvation. He is my God, and I will praise him, my father's God, and I will exalt him." (Ex. 15:1-2)

The Israelites crossed the Red Sea on dry land. The Egyptian army, however, was destroyed as the sea's water returned and drowned them. Moses had much to be grateful for. Hindsight proved that God keeps His promises.

✟ There are forty years yet to come of wandering and complaining. Do the Israelites' future mistakes and lack of faith make this song any less meaningful to God?

✟ The Israelites did not know what their trek to the Promised Land entailed. If you had foresight concerning your own life, what would you like to see in your future?

✟ How can you make God your song? What refrain would you want to repeat throughout the song?

JOURNAL: JOHN 2:1-11 ARE YOUR NEEDS IMPORTANT TO GOD? HOW DO YOU KNOW?

Sing A New Song #8

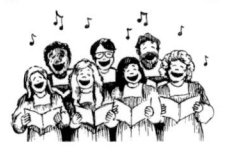

Sing to the LORD a new song, his praise from the ends of the earth, you who go down to the sea, and all that is in it, you islands, and all who live in them. (Isa. 42:10)

☦ Just where does the earth end? What insight can you glean from the inclusive term "ends of the earth"?

☦ How far is the east from the west? Do they ever meet? Why not use the phrase "as far as the north is from the south"?

☦ What does the phrase, "No man is an island," mean to you?

☦ Isaiah 42:16 continues, *I will lead the blind by ways they have not known, along unfamiliar paths I will guide them; I will turn the darkness into light before them and make the rough places smooth. These are the things I will do; I will not forsake them.* Chronic illness is certainly an unfamiliar path. What promises does God give you in this verse? Do they comfort you? If not, why not?

JOURNAL: PS. 100 FIND 6 REASONS TO PRAISE THE LORD.

Moses: Man of Song #9

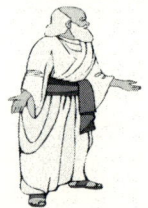

¹⁹Now write down for yourselves this song and teach it to the Israelites and have them sing it, so that it may be a witness for me against them. ²⁰When I have brought them into the land flowing with milk and honey, the land I promised on oath to their forefathers, and when they eat their fill and thrive, they will turn to other gods and worship them, rejecting me and breaking my covenant." (Deut. 31:19-20)

✝ God gave His people a song to remember His past victories and their future broken promises. (Read the song in Deut. 32.) Why do you think God would have Moses record a song that foretold the Israelite's failures?

✝ Since the Israelites will not follow after God's ways nor continue to worship Him after they enter the Promised Land, why does God give them the land?

✝ Are you inspired or discouraged by God's knowledge of your future weaknesses and failures? Why?

JOURNAL: JAMES 5:13-16 IS THIS PASSAGE A RECIPE FOR HEALING? IF YOU DO ALL THAT IT SAYS, DOES THAT MAKE YOU A PERFECT CHRISTIAN? WHY?

Sing A New Song #9

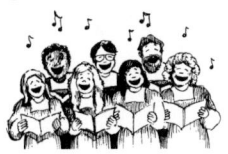

¹⁹*Speak to one another with psalms, hymns and spiritual songs. Sing and make music in your heart to the Lord,* ²⁰*always giving thanks to God the Father for everything, in the name of our Lord Jesus Christ.* (Eph. 5:19-20)

☦ Is there any difference between "psalms," "hymns," and "spiritual songs"? Explain.

☦ What do you have to be thankful for right this minute? List at least 3 things and sing a song of gratitude.

☦ Eph. 3:20 states, **Now to him who is able to do immeasurably more than all we ask or imagine, according to his power that is at work within us.** How is God's power working within you today?

☦ How is God's power revealed through your illness?

☦ Do you need to praise God when you're sick? Why?

JOURNAL: REV. 5:9-14 IS CHRIST WORTHY? ARE YOU? WHY?

Moses: Man of Song #10

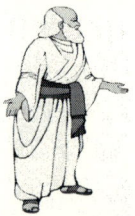

³⁰Moses recited the words of this song from beginning to end in the hearing of the whole assembly of Israel: ¹"Listen, O heavens, and I will speak; hear, O earth, the words of my mouth." (Deut. 31:30, 32:1)

While Moses wandered in the wilderness for forty years, he recorded God's laws that established the Jewish religion. All the people who left Egypt were dead and only their children remained. These forty years in the desert revealed a true heart change in Moses. He no longer asked God to "send someone else" but accepted his responsibilities.

☦ Which event, or events, do you think were the most significant in changing Moses' "tune"? Explain.

☦ God demanded that Moses and Joshua write down His words in song so that the Israelites would remember His signs, miracles, and works. Journaling is Biblical! Does knowing this make journaling more important to you? If yes, why? If not, why not?

☦ What life event changed your tune from noise to joy?

JOURNAL: PS. 121 WHERE CAN YOU FIND HELP WHEN YOU'RE IN TROUBLE?

Sing A New Song #10

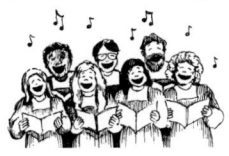

Seven angels with harps, *³...sang the song of Moses the servant of God and the song of the Lamb: 'Great and marvelous are your deeds, Lord God Almighty. Just and true are your ways, King of the ages. ⁴Who will not fear you, O Lord, and bring glory to your name? For you alone are holy. All nations will come and worship before you, for your righteous acts have been revealed.'* (Rev. 15:3-4)

The Bible's written message ends with the book of Revelations, and through it the Holy Spirit continues to teach, rebuke, encourage and inspire us. When we believers arrive in Heaven, we'll hear Moses' song, and yet more thrilling, we'll hear the song of the Lamb, Jesus Christ.

☥ Jesus revealed the righteous acts of God. Explain how.

☥ What have you learned about God from Moses' life?

☥ Your choice in life's circumstances is to either make a loud noise over your difficulties or to sing a new song of gratitude and thanksgiving. What is your response?

JOURNAL: PS. 119:1-11 WHAT NOUNS ARE USED TO DESCRIBE THE DIFFERENT FACETS OF GOD'S WORD?

CHAPTER THREE

Cursed by Enemies or Blessed by God

Nehemiah was a man of action who took God's commands seriously, and was intent that other Jews should also. He was not discouraged by impossible tasks nor strutting enemies. He was undeterred from God's call to rebuild the wall surrounding Jerusalem that had been left in rubble after the Babylonian invasion.

Nehemiah understood the intrigues and politics of both the Persian royal court and of the petty despots who ruled the territory adjacent to Israel: Sanballat, Governor of Samaria, Tobiah, Governor of Transjordan, and Geshem, controller of vast areas from northeast Egypt to northern Arabia & Southern Palestine. These spiteful, narrow-minded tyrants continually harassed Nehemiah and his building efforts. They threatened his life, sent false reports back to the Persian king, and tried to trick him with false prophets. They attempted to cause discord and discouragement among the Jewish workers as they bullied, taunted and cursed them. Every action by these men was designed to intimidate Nehemiah, and yet he overcame every distraction and let nothing stand in his way from completing the mission God called him to.

Nehemiah could have hurled curses and reviled those who plagued him. Instead, he remained focused on what was really important—his relationship with God and the work He had given him to do. Nehemiah models for us God's effective formula for responding to crises: pray first, wait for God's timing, then take action.

Practical Nehemiah: Blessed of God #1

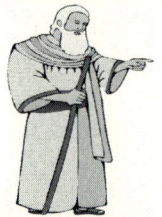

Nehemiah prayed, *"O Lord, let your ear be attentive to the prayer of this your servant and to the prayer of your servants who delight in revering your name. Give your servant success today by granting him favor in the presence of this man..."* Nehemiah was cupbearer to the king of Persia, Artaxerxes. (Neh. 1:11a)

When Nehemiah heard of Jerusalem's ruin, he wept, mourned, fasted, and prayed night and day, confessing his nation's disobedience, his own sinfulness, and God's promise to return the Jews to Jerusalem. During this time, Nehemiah prepared himself to face Artaxerxes by going to God and by planning ahead of time what he should say.

✞ What could you ask the King of Heaven to allow you to do that would not be for personal gain?

✞ King Artaxerxes had life and death control over Nehemiah. How is your life controlled by your illness?

✞ Is pain negotiable with healthcare professionals, with your surroundings, with medications, with God? Explain.

JOURNAL: PS. 77 ON WHOM SHOULD YOU MEDITATE? WHY?

Cursed or Blessed #1

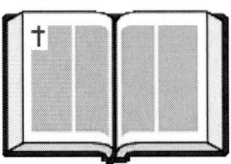

Blessed is he who has regard for the weak; the LORD delivers him in times of trouble. (Ps. 41:1)

Chronic illness tires and weakens us. David tells us, **He [God] rescued me from my powerful enemy, from my foes, who were too strong for me.** (Ps. 18:17)

☦ Does your physical illness make you feel frail spiritually, emotionally, or mentally? How does God deliver you when you feel this way?

☦ Are you sick and tired of being sick and tired? What's one practical action you can take today to break this cycle of discouragement?

☦ When do you feel strong in spite of your illness? If infrequently or never, read Psalm 18.

☦ How do you encourage other people with chronic illness?

JOURNAL: I COR. 13 REPLACE "LOVE" AND "IT" IN VS. 4-7 WITH "JESUS." JESUS IS THE DEFINITION OF LOVE. NOW USE YOUR NAME. HOW CAN YOUR ACTIONS DISPLAY THIS KIND OF LOVE?

Practical Nehemiah: Blessed of God #2

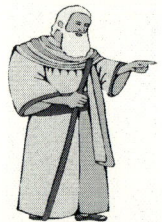

¹...I took the wine and gave it to the king. I had not been sad in his presence before; ²so the king asked me, "Why does your face look so sad when you are not ill? This can be nothing but sadness of heart." I was very much afraid, ⁴...Then I prayed to the God of heaven, ⁵and I answered the king..." (Neh. 2:1b, 2, 4b, 5a)

Daily intimacy with the King offered no protection for Nehemiah. Court protocol required that the King must speak first before being spoken to. Note that Nehemiah prayed, then he spoke.

✞ God called Nehemiah to a dangerous work, even before he left home. Are you in a threatening situation?

✞ Have you spoken before you thought things through and gotten yourself in trouble? What happened?

✞ What has caused you "sadness of heart"?

JOURNAL: PS. 107:1-16 WHAT KIND OF TROUBLE CAN YOU GET INTO WHEN YOU REBEL AGAINST GOD? ONCE YOU RECOGNIZE YOUR SIN, HOW DOES GOD RESPOND WHEN YOU CRY OUT TO HIM?

Cursed or Blessed #2

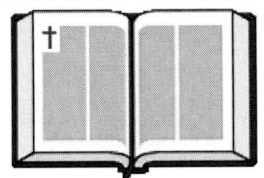

Blessed are those who have learned to acclaim you, who walk in the light of your presence, O LORD. (Ps. 89:15)

Blessed (happy, fortunate, to be envied) are the people who know the joyful sound [who understand and appreciate the spiritual blessings symbolized by the feasts]; they walk, O Lord, in the light and favor of Your countenance! (Ps. 89:15 The Amplified Bible)

✞ What does the phrase, "walk in the light of God's presence," mean to you?

✞ How and when did you learn to praise God?

✞ Where do you worship God most frequently: at church, at home, in the car, in the doctor's office? Why there?

✞ Have you ever found yourself worshipping God unexpectedly? If so, when? If not, why not?

JOURNAL: JOHN 17:6-19 HOW CAN YOU USE THIS EXAMPLE OF JESUS INTERCEDING FOR THE DISCIPLES IN YOUR OWN PRAYER LIFE?

Practical Nehemiah: Blessed of God #3

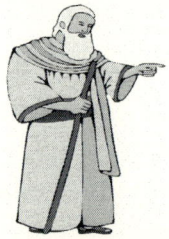

¹⁷Then I said to them, "You see the trouble we are in: Jerusalem lies in ruins, and its gates have been burned with fire. Come, let us rebuild the wall of Jerusalem, and we will no longer be in disgrace." ¹⁸I also told them about the gracious hand of my God upon me... (Neh. 2:17-18a)

God gave Nehemiah courage to stand before a conquered, people and give them hope. **They replied, "Let us start rebuilding." So they began this good work.** (Neh. 2:18b) Meanwhile, **When Sanballat the Horonite and Tobiah the Ammonite official heard about this, they were very much disturbed that someone had come to promote the welfare of the Israelites.** (Neh. 2:10)

✞ When you interact with a health care provider, do you feel courageous like Nehemiah, disheartened like an Israelite, or skeptical like an official? Why is that?

✞ Nehemiah started this project with the assurance that God would see it finished. Nehemiah did not listen to his enemies or their slander. When beginning a new medical treatment, what is your attitude? Does it help?

JOURNAL: PS. 122 WHAT GIVES YOU A SENSE OF PEACE? WHY?

Cursed or Blessed #3

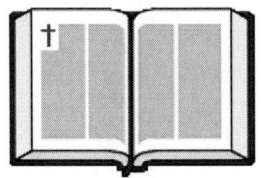

²⁷Let them know that it is your hand, that you, O LORD, have done it. ²⁸They may curse, but you will bless; when they attack they will be put to shame, but your servant will rejoice. (Ps. 109:27-28)

Though God did not cause your illness, He will not waste it either. Cursing your situation amplifies your struggles, blessing God lifts your spirit above your circumstances.

✝ How can knowing that God allows your suffering be an encouragement? If it is not, think again.

✝ If God allows pain so that He may bless you, what changes do you need to make in your attitude toward your illness?

✝ Is there any shame attached to your illness? If so, how do you deal with it? If not, explain.

✝ How can you "rejoice" when non-supportive, critical people are in your life?

JOURNAL: PS. 91 HOW CAN YOU APPLY THESE WORDS OF GOD'S PROTECTION TO YOUR LIFE TODAY?

Practical Nehemiah: Blessed of God #4

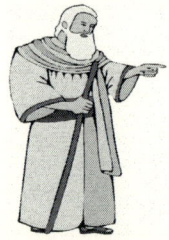

But when Sanballat, Tobiah, and Geshem, heard about the work, [19]...*they mocked and ridiculed us. "What is this you are doing?"... "Are you rebelling against the king?"* [20]*I answered them by saying, "The God of heaven will give us success. We his servants will start rebuilding, but as for you, you have no share in Jerusalem or any claim or historic right to it."* (Neh. 2:19b-20)

✟ Nehemiah was not deflected by others' criticism. How do you respond to critical remarks?

✟ Is pain your enemy or is it God's plan for accomplishing spiritual intimacy? Explain.

✟ Who around you disbelieves, misunderstands, or does not acknowledge your health crisis? What can you do?

✟ List three statements that would educate naysayers about your health condition.

JOURNAL: PS. 111 HOW DO YOU RECALL GOD'S GOOD DEEDS?

Cursed or Blessed #4

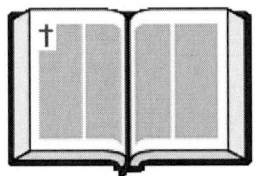

⁷Be at rest once more, O my soul, for the LORD has been good to you. ⁸For you, O LORD, have delivered my soul from death, my eyes from tears, my feet from stumbling, ⁹that I may walk before the LORD in the land of the living. (Ps.116:7-9)

✞ What time of day does your body rest? For how long? When does your spirit and soul rest? If never, how can you find respite for your weariness?

✞ In what event has God taken your tears of sorrow and pain and blessed you in spite of yourself?

✞ How has God been good to you this week? What do you have to be thankful for today?

✞ Since 90% of chronic illness is invisible, do you ever feel as if no one understands your suffering? How does this Scripture, Ps. 116:7-9, offer you hope?

JOURNAL: 2 THESS. 1:1-12 HOW HAS YOUR ILLNESS ENCOURAGED PERSEVERANCE? HOW HAS JESUS BEEN REVEALED THROUGH YOUR TRIALS?

Practical Nehemiah: Blessed of God #5

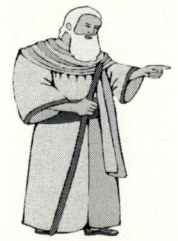

Sanballat spoke in the presence of his associates and the army of Samaria, *²"...What are those feeble Jews doing? Will they restore their wall? Will they offer sacrifices? Will they finish in a day? Can they bring the stones back to life from those heaps of rubble-- burned as they are?"* [Nehemiah responded] *⁴"Hear us, O our God, for we are despised. Turn their insults back on their own heads. Give them over as plunder in a land of captivity. ⁵Do not cover up their guilt or blot out their sins from your sight, for they have thrown insults in the face of the builders."* (Neh. 4:2b, 4-5)

Nehemiah did not confront his adversaries. Instead, he took their insults to God and requested that God wreak His vengeance upon them.

✞ What's your response to ill-informed people: ignore them, change the topic, educate them, be sarcastic, point out their ignorance, leave the room? Why?

✞ When have you prayed before speaking? Did it help the situation? How? If it did not, why not?

JOURNAL: JOHN 8:1-11 WHAT IS GOD'S OPINION ABOUT JUDGING OTHERS? CAN YOU LIVE THIS WAY?

Cursed or Blessed #5

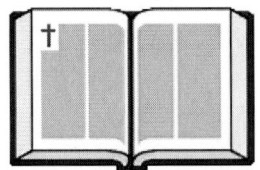

²⁷But I tell you who hear me: Love your enemies, do good to those who hate you, ²⁸bless those who curse you, pray for those who mistreat you. (Luke 6:27-28)

✝ Your chronic illness can become an enemy that wreaks havoc with your life, allowing you to shake your fist at God, to be angry about your circumstances, and to mismanage your relationships. How can these words of Jesus provide you with a strategy for dealing with your pain?

✝ Medical support is extremely important for those of us who have chronic pain. What do you think about your medical resources? No one listens to me. My doctor is sympathetic. I work with a medical team intent on improving my health. I've been sent to a psychiatrist. I am lost in a sea of paperwork. How does this support, or lack thereof, make you feel? What can you do about it?

✝ Why would praying for your thorns, that is your daily pain, make the rose of living smell sweeter? Do you?

JOURNAL: MARK 2:1-12 WHAT SPIRITUAL HEALING HAVE YOU EXPERIENCED? PHYSICAL HEALING? EMOTIONAL HEALING? IS IT ENOUGH?

Practical Nehemiah: Blessed of God #6

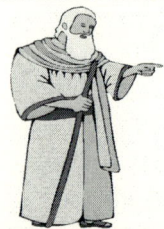

⁸They all plotted together to come and fight against Jerusalem and stir up trouble against it. ⁹But we prayed to our God and posted a guard day and night to meet this threat. (Neh. 4:8-9)

Nehemiah met each circumstance with the same solution: pray then proceed. His enemies were scheming men of deceit. Their goal was to discredit Nehemiah and maintain their power, keeping Jerusalem weak and its people in fear. Nehemiah's goal, on the other hand, focused on the task God had set for him, and he let nothing stand in his way.

☦ Nehemiah's constant prayers and God's provision invigorated the workers. What are you praying for?

☦ How does prayer for others help you through your own difficult circumstances? If you don't pray for others, how can you begin this blessing-filled habit?

☦ Nehemiah's enemies used gossip and slander to spread discord among the people. How do you avoid these traps?

JOURNAL: PS. 25 WHAT LESSONS DO YOU STILL NEED TO LEARN ABOUT GOD? ABOUT YOUR HEALTH?

Cursed or Blessed #6

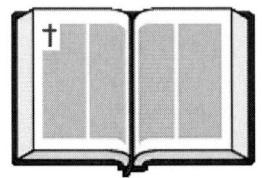

Jesus said, *"Father, if you are willing, take this cup from me; yet not my will, but yours be done."* (Luke 22:42)

The night of Jesus' arrest, He prayed fervently to His Heavenly Father that there would be another way to provide salvation for mankind. There was no other way but to go to the cross. So Jesus did.

✝ When you say, "not my will, but yours be done" to God, what do *you* mean?

✝ Have you released your will in the matter of your chronic illness and accepted that this is the way your life's journey will be? If so, how do you feel spiritually and emotionally? If not, in what traps are you entangled?

✝ Have you ever asked for prayer from the elders of your church, gone to a healing service, or asked friends to pray for your healing? If so, how has God answered your spiritual efforts? If you have not asked for prayer, "should" you? Why?

JOURNAL: LUKE 18:1-8 HOW IS GOD DIFFERENT FROM THIS JUDGE? CAN GOD BE MANIPULATED WITH PRAYER? DO YOU EVER TRY? WHAT HAPPENS?

Practical Nehemiah: Blessed of God #7

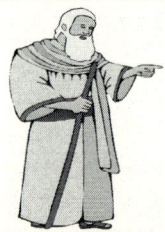

¹¹Also our enemies said, "Before they know it or see us, we will be right there among them and will kill them and put an end to the work." ¹⁴After I looked things over, I stood up and said to the nobles, the officials and the rest of the people, "Don't be afraid of them. Remember the Lord, who is great and awesome..." (Neh. 4:11, 14a)

Nehemiah had the people working with a spear in one hand and building materials in the other. **When our enemies heard that we were aware of their plot and that God had frustrated it, we all returned to the wall, each to his own work.** (Neh. 4:15)

✢ Do you do things one-at-a-time or multi-task? How has your illness compromised your abilities?

✢ Consider how Satan piles on guilt using your illness as a catalyst. How can you discredit his influence?

✢ Which is harder for you: external disapproval or internal anxiety? Explain.

JOURNAL: JOHN 14:15-27 WHEN DO YOU EXPERIENCE THE COUNSELOR JESUS SPEAKS OF? EXPLAIN.

Cursed or Blessed #7

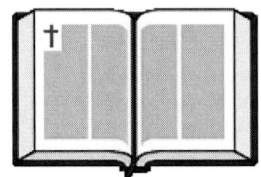

Bless those who persecute you; bless and do not curse. (Rom. 12:14 NIV)

Blessed and happy and enviably fortunate and spiritually prosperous (in the state in which the born-again child of God enjoys and finds satisfaction in God's favor and salvation, regardless of his outward conditions) are those who are persecuted for righteousness' sake (for being and doing right), for theirs is the kingdom of heaven! (Matt. 5:10 AMP)

✞ Matt. 5:10 above defines the term of being "spiritually prosperous." What does this state of being look like in your life?

✞ Do you expect sympathy from others? Do you view your illness as a curse? How can you adjust your attitude so that you can put into practice more positive behaviors?

✞ How has your illness forced you to change your lifestyle? Has this change been positive? What negative factors has this change brought? What behavior will help you deal with your negative thoughts?

JOURNAL: PS. 23 HOW DOES GOD CARE FOR YOU?

Practical Nehemiah: Blessed of God #8

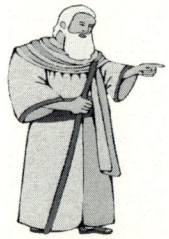

¹¹But I said, "Should a man like me run away? Or should one like me go into the temple to save his life? I will not go!" ¹²I realized that God had not sent him, but that he had prophesied against me because Tobiah and Sanballat had hired him. (Neh. 6:11-12)

A false prophet tried to talk Nehemiah into hiding himself in the temple so that he would not be killed at night in his bed. But astute Nehemiah determined that the prophet *...had been hired to intimidate me so that I would commit a sin by doing this, and then they would give me a bad name to discredit me.* (Neh. 6:13b)

☦ Have you ever felt like running away? When? Why?

☦ If you ran away now, where would you go? Why?

☦ Have you ever been tempted to hide from the work God's planned for you? How did you overcome the temptation? If you did not, what can you do now?

JOURNAL: MATT. 11:25-30 WHAT ARE YOUR CURRENT BURDENS? HOW CAN JESUS' YOLK HELP? CAN HIS YOLK EVER HINDER YOU? HOW?

Cursed or Blessed #8

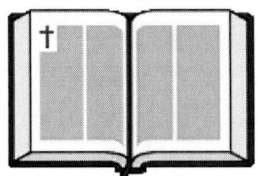

⁹With the tongue we praise our Lord and Father, and with it we curse men, who have been made in God's likeness. ¹⁰Out of the same mouth come praise and cursing. My brothers, this should not be. (James 3:9-10)

✝ What is your tongue created to do?

✝ Does cursing or speaking ill of people offend God? Explain.

✝ As illness forces you to modify your life-style, do you blame God or others for making your life difficult? How do you fall into this trap? What can you do to escape?

✝ Are circumstances or relationships more vital to God?

✝ Which do you do more often? Complain to God about your situation or praise Him for your relationships?

JOURNAL: I COR. 4:1-7 DO YOU JUDGE OTHER PEOPLE? DO YOU FEAR THAT OTHERS ARE JUDGING YOU? HOW DOES THAT MAKE YOU FEEL?

Practical Nehemiah: Blessed of God #9

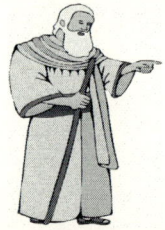

¹⁵So the wall was completed on the twenty-fifth of Elul, in fifty-two days. ¹⁶When all our enemies heard about this, all the surrounding nations were afraid and lost their self-confidence, because they realized that this work had been done with the help of our God. (Neh. 6:15-16)

Absolutely amazing! In 52 days, impassable rubble was cleared, stones were found, carried and aligned, gates were built and set in place. The Jerusalem wall, more than half a football field high, was completed in seven weeks. By trusting in God and not being distracted by his enemies, Nehemiah finished his wall-building project in record time.

☦ Viewing your illness as a lifetime project, how can you silence discouragement, fear, and despair?

☦ What one area in your life needs to be cleared of rubble?

☦ Through the course of your illness, what amazing event has happened to reveal God's hand in your life?

JOURNAL: EPH. 1:1-14 WHAT SPIRITUAL BLESSINGS DO YOU HAVE IN CHRIST? LIST THEM.

Cursed or Blessed #9

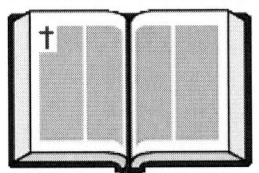

Do not repay evil with evil or insult with insult, but with blessing, because to this you were called so that you may inherit a blessing. (1 Peter 3:9)

✞ Do you allow yourself to be offended by thoughtless people who do not understand your chronic condition? Why? If not, how do you handle people's insensitivity?

✞ How can you bless an insulting person? Should you?

✞ Some people consider your illness to be a curse. If that is so, do you agree with any of these statements? I am cursed. It's my bad luck. Satan is hounding me. God is punishing me. I'm not taking good care of myself. I am sick due to generational sin. If you disagree with any or all of these statements, then why are you ill?

✞ Do you hold grudges? What promise of God's can you claim to free yourself from this negative behavior? Who can you contact right now to ask forgiveness from and to be a blessing to?

JOURNAL: MATT. 18:21-35 DO YOU OFFER FORGIVENESS TO OTHERS? WHY IS FORGIVENESS IMPORTANT?

Practical Nehemiah: Blessed of God #10

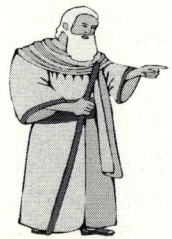

Nehemiah angrily asked the merchants, *²¹"Why do you spend the night by the wall? If you do this again, I will lay hands on you." From that time on they no longer came on the Sabbath. ²²Then I commanded the Levites to purify themselves and go and guard the gates in order to keep the Sabbath day holy. "Remember me for this also, O my God, and show mercy to me according to your great love."* (Neh. 13:21-22)

Nehemiah returned to Persia to report his work's completion. The people of Jerusalem, however, fell back into old behavior patterns not pleasing to God. Nehemiah, therefore, went back to the city to cleanse the people of pagan practices.

☦ How do you keep the Sabbath day holy?

☦ What decision have you made recently that was Spirit led? If none, what is intruding between you and God?

☦ Name one important thing you learned from Nehemiah.

JOURNAL: JOHN 16:5-15 WHAT DOES THE HOLY SPIRIT OFFER YOU EVERY MOMENT OF YOUR LIFE?

Cursed or Blessed #10

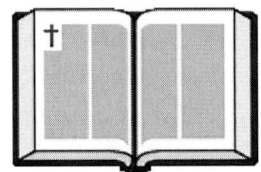

But in your hearts set apart Christ as Lord. Always be prepared to give an answer to everyone who asks you to give the reason for the hope that you have. But do this with gentleness and respect, (1Peter 3:15)

☦ Do you ever feel compelled to explain your behavior in light of your pain? If so, why? If not, why not?

☦ Do you have any relationships where you feel misunderstood, apologetic, or ashamed? Explain.

☦ When you do <u>not</u> act like a "good Christian," do people question your authenticity? Do you? Why?

☦ Do your conversations continually include illness related up-dates? Does your illness overshadow the blessings in your life? If so, what new habit do you need to practice?

☦ What circumstances or relationships give you hope?

JOURNAL: PS. 71 DOES YOUR ILLNESS MAKE YOU FEEL OLD? HOW DOES THIS PSALM ENCOURAGE YOU?

CHAPTER FOUR

Worldly Cares or Heavenly Promises

Paul was raised, and grew to manhood, as a strict, Pharisitical Jew, meaning that outwardly he followed Moses' Law to the letter. God, however, got Paul's attention on the road to Damascus, and Paul became a fanatic follower of Jesus Christ. He spoke the message of Salvation to the non-Jewish world, the Gentiles.

Paul certainly had every reason for a world-weary attitude. In Corinthians he recounts, [24]*Five times I received from the Jews the forty lashes minus one.* [25]*Three times I was beaten with rods, once I was stoned, three times I was shipwrecked, I spent a night and a day in the open sea,* [26]*I have been constantly on the move. I have been in danger from rivers, in danger from bandits, in danger from my own countrymen, in danger from Gentiles; in danger in the city, in danger in the country, in danger at sea; and in danger from false brothers.* [27]*I have labored and toiled and have often gone without sleep; I have known hunger and thirst and have often gone without food; I have been cold and naked.* (2 Cor.11: 24-27)

And how did Paul respond to his hardships? *I press on toward the goal to win the prize for which God has called me heavenward in Christ Jesus.* (Phil. 3:14)

Paul's afflictions enabled him to encourage the followers of Christ to focus on their higher calling and not to focus on their current suffering. His spiritual walk models for us a heavenly-focus rather than an earthly perspective of physical suffering, changing circumstances, and damaged relationships.

Paul: Heavenly Minded #1

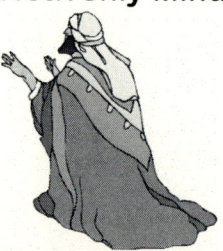

Therefore, my brothers, I want you to know that through Jesus the forgiveness of sins is proclaimed to you. (Acts 13:38)

On the road to Damascus, Paul discovered first hand the forgiveness of Jesus Christ. Paul set out to imprison all Christians, but Jesus stepped into his life, blinded him with His glory, returned his sight in three days, and sent him out to preach the Good News of Christ to the Gentile world.

☦ What did you experience when you first met Jesus?

☦ How uncomfortable is it for you to share your Salvation story of Jesus Christ with others? Explain.

☦ When have you shared the Good News of Salvation with anyone? How did he or she respond? How did you feel? If you have never shared the Gospel, why not?

☦ Does your illness help or hinder your sharing the Gospel?

JOURNAL: PS. 146 WHY DO YOU HOPE IN THE LORD?

Heavenly Promises #1

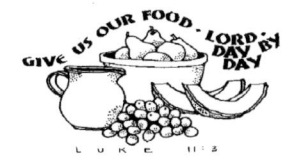

For no matter how many promises God has made, they are "Yes" in Christ. And so through him the "Amen" is spoken by us to the glory of God. (2 Cor.1:20)

"Amen!" means "It is true!" or "So be it!" spoken by the believer acknowledging that the words said are utterly authentic.

✟ What are the most important promises God has made to you? How many will He keep? How do you know?

✟ What does the "Yes in Christ!" mean to you?

✟ What does saying "Amen!" mean to you?

✟ When do you declare "Amen!": at the end of saying grace, at the end of speaking a prayer, during church service, in the middle of a sermon, in bed at the beginning/end of the day, in general conversation? Which of these occasions are appropriate? When is it inappropriate to say, "Amen"? Why?

JOURNAL: PS. 1 WHEN DO YOU RECOGNIZE YOU ARE BLESSED? HOW DO YOU RESPOND?

Paul: Heavenly Minded #2

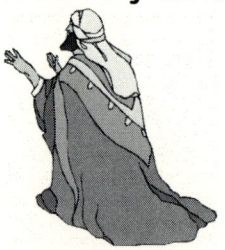

For the Lord himself will come down from heaven, with a loud command, with the voice of the archangel and with the trumpet call of God, and the dead in Christ will rise first. (1 Thess. 4:16)

Paul certainly understood "dead" in terms of experience. He was stoned and left for dead by irate Jews. Yet he got up and set off for Derbe the next day. (Acts. 14:19-20)

✞ How can you prepare for Christ's promised return?

✞ In the Scripture above, how does Paul's assurance to the Thessalonians better prepare you for your own death? If it does not, why not?

✞ Do you know anyone who has died of your illness? How do you cope with this knowledge? Has anyone recovered or had improved symptoms? How does that make you feel?

JOURNAL: JOHN 14:1-14 DOES KNOWING YOU WILL GO TO HEAVEN RELIEVE YOUR CONCERNS HERE ON EARTH? HOW? IF NOT, WHY NOT?

Heavenly Promises #2

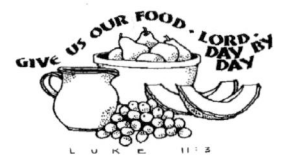

Since we have these promises, dear friends, let us purify ourselves from everything that contaminates body and spirit, perfecting holiness out of reverence for God. (2 Cor. 7:1)

☦ What contaminates your body? Your spirit? Your mind?

☦ Does your illness cause you to feel unclean or impure? Why? What can you do to change your feelings? If you never feel unclean before God, why not?

☦ What do you do to show reverence to God? Do your actions make you holy? Explain.

☦ 1 Peter 1:15-16 exhorts the importance of holiness, *^{15}But just as he who called you is holy, so be holy in all you do; ^{16} for it is written: "Be holy, because I am holy."* We are to reflect God's holiness. You cannot make yourself like God, so how can you be holy? When God looks at your heart, does he see you or Jesus? Why is this so? Must you do anything to change God's view?

JOURNAL: MATT. 13:44-51 WHAT DOES THE KINGDOM OF HEAVEN LOOK LIKE HERE ON EARTH?

Paul: Heavenly Minded #3

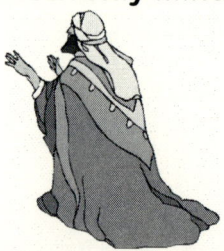

To keep me from becoming conceited because of these surpassingly great revelations, there was given me a thorn in my flesh, a messenger of Satan, to torment me. (2 Cor. 12:7)

Paul was not a strong, robust man even though he traveled extensively. After he prayed three times to be relieved of his physical suffering, God answered, *My grace is sufficient for you, for my power is made perfect in weakness.* Paul accepted God's, "No!" by claiming, *Therefore I will boast all the more gladly about my weaknesses, so that Christ's power may rest on me."* (2 Cor. 12:9)

✞ What is your "thorn in the flesh"? How does it torment you?

✞ How can your weakness of flesh be of any use to God?

✞ How does your suffering serve a higher purpose? Is this comforting? Explain.

JOURNAL: 2 COR. 4 WHAT ARE YOUR EARTHLY TROUBLES? DOES GOD'S LOVE DIMINISH YOUR SUFFERING? EXPLAIN.

Heavenly Promises #3

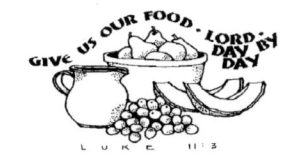

He redeemed us in order that the blessing given to Abraham might come to the Gentiles through Christ Jesus, so that by faith we might receive the promise of the Spirit. (Gal. 3:14)

Jewish religion claims Abraham as the father of the Jews (Rom. 4:16). Paul declared that since Abraham came before the Law of Moses, Gentiles were not bound by the Law, and so were also entitled to the promise of Christ's Salvation.

☦ God chose the Jews through whom would come the Savior of the world. With all the rituals the Jews bound themselves to, they forgot why they were God's chosen people. You are also chosen. When you are in pain, what promises of God do you forget to claim?

☦ Once you have received Jesus as your personal Savior, you are infused with the Holy Spirit. Do you access or deny His power when you are in pain?

☦ What ways can you avail yourself of God's power?

JOURNAL: JAMES 1:1-12 WHEN HAVE YOU PERSEVERED IN A ILLNESS CRISIS AND BEEN BLESSED?

Paul: Heavenly Minded #4

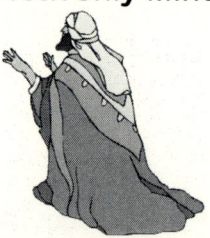

This girl followed Paul and the rest of us, shouting, "These men are servants of the Most High God, who are telling you the way to be saved." (Acts 16:17)

A slave girl, who predicted the future, made this declaration day after day until Paul cast the demon out of her. Because of this action, her owners brought Paul before the authorities and had him severely flogged.

✞ Was the slave girl's declaration a nuisance, a hindrance, a benefit, a contest, or an antagonism to Paul? Explain.

✞ The girl's owners resisted the Gospel message because it cost them financially. Does your financial situation obstruct or encourage you from sharing or supporting the spread of the Gospel? How?

✞ Have you been "flogged" by accusations that you are making up symptoms so that you need a psychiatrist instead of a medical doctor? How does/did that make you feel? What can you do about such ignorant opinions?

JOURNAL: JOHN 15:12-27 DO YOU SHOW LOVE TO OTHERS WHEN THEY ARE NOT SO LOVING? HOW?

Heavenly Promises #4

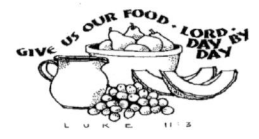

Praise be to the God and Father of our Lord Jesus Christ, who has blessed us in the heavenly realms with every spiritual blessing in Christ. (Eph. 1:3)

- ✞ When you hear the term "blessing" what comes to mind: experiencing answered prayer, coming into possession of some thing, participating in an event with a positive outcome, having a moving spiritual experience? Explain.

- ✞ Read Eph. 1:4-9 to discover "every spiritual blessing" you have in Christ. Find at least seven spiritual blessings and list them.

- ✞ Which spiritual blessings comfort you? Why?

- ✞ Can you compare spiritual blessings to physical blessings? Explain.

- ✞ How does the knowledge that God loves and blesses you help you to love and bless others? Why?

JOURNAL: I JOHN 4:7-21 DO YOU LIVE YOUR LIFE IN LOVE?

Paul: Heavenly Minded #5

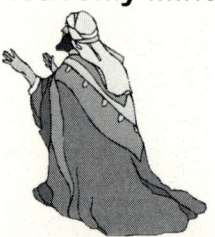

But the Scripture declares that the whole world is a prisoner of sin, so that what was promised, being given through faith in Jesus Christ, might be given to those who believe. (Gal. 3:22)

After the earlier flogging, Paul was imprisoned and his feet bound in stocks. When an earthquake struck at midnight, he was praying and singing hymns. Because he did not try to escape, the jailer took Paul into his home, and he and his whole household were saved. (Acts 16:25-31)

☦ The jailer's conversion implies that the circumstances of flogging and imprisonment were for God's purpose. Looking at your own circumstances, can you identify God's purpose for you? How does that make you feel?

☦ Does your illness make you feel like a prisoner? What wisdom does this story offer you when faced with difficult times?

☦ Is it hard to pray or sing in the midst of pain? Why?

JOURNAL: MATT. 6:25-34 HOW CAN YOU RELEASE YOUR WORRIES OVER SOME OF THE "THINGS" GOD HAS PROMISED TO TAKE CARE OF?

Heavenly Promises #5

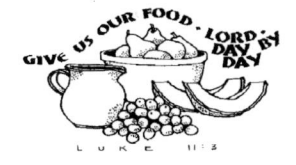

And you also were included in Christ when you heard the word of truth, the gospel of your salvation. Having believed, you were marked in him with a seal, the promised Holy Spirit, (Eph. 1:13)

The phrase, "marked… with a seal" signifies ownership. In the spiritual world you are either God's or Satan's. Being God's child does not mean you have to be perfect, but rather that He chose you before time began and marked you with something permanent—His seal, the Holy Spirit.

✝ How does knowing that you are sealed for all eternity as God's chosen child give you comfort? If it does not, why not?

✝ Does going to church mark you as God's child? Why do you think so?

✝ Why would God choose you with your body so broken?

✝ Do you sense the Holy Spirit's presence? Explain.

JOURNAL: JOHN 16:22-33 CAN GRIEF TURN TO JOY? HOW?

Paul: Heavenly Minded #6

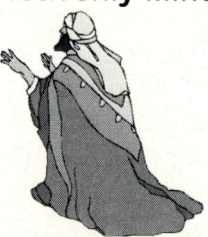

¹⁴Then he said: "The God of our fathers has chosen you to know his will and to see the Righteous One and to hear words from his mouth. ¹⁵You will be his witness to all men of what you have seen and heard." (Acts 22:14-15)

Returning to Jerusalem, Paul witnessed in the temple and concluded: *Then the Lord said to me, 'Go; I will send you far away to the Gentiles.'* (Acts 22:21) The Jews became incensed and rioted. Messiah for the Gentiles, or non-Jew was unthinkable.

☦ Since you are chosen by God, what do you know about His will for you?

☦ To whom do you have the opportunity to witness? Do you? Explain.

☦ Who has authority over your medical decisions: you, your doctor, your family, a care-giver, an insurance company, medical personnel? How do you feel about it?

JOURNAL: PS. 56 WHAT CAUSES STRESS IN YOUR LIFE? CAN WHAT YOU KNOW ABOUT GOD RELIEVE THIS STRESS? HOW?

Heavenly Promises #6

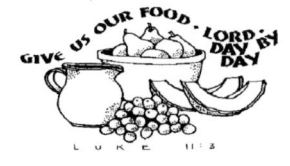

⁸ For it is by grace you have been saved, through faith--and this not from yourselves, it is the gift of God-- ⁹ not by works, so that no one can boast. (Eph 2:8-9)

✞ Whose grace has saved you?

✞ Where does your faith come from? What other gifts has God given you besides faith and salvation?

✞ What does the term "not by works" mean to you?

✞ Paul states in 1 Cor 1:31, **Therefore, as it is written: "Let him who boasts boast in the Lord."** What do you have to boast about? If nothing, think again.

✞ Does your illness affect your ability to boast in the Lord? How? If not, how do you overcome the "dailyness" of chronic pain and fatigue?

JOURNAL: ROM. 12:9-21 HERE'S A LIST OF CHRISTIAN BEHAVIORS. CAN YOU PERFORM THEM ALL? WHICH ONES? WHO ACCOMPLISHES THE REST?

Paul: Heavenly Minded #7

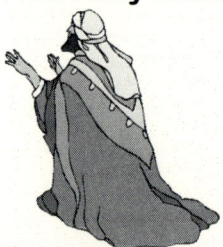

I press on toward the goal to win the prize for which God has called me heavenward in Christ Jesus. (Phil. 3:14)

Accosted by rioting Jews in the synagogue, Paul was whisked away by Roman soldiers with orders to flog then question him. (Acts 22:24) Paul declared himself a Roman citizen, innocent until proven guilty. In so stating, however, he would have to be taken to Rome, an arduous journey, and there stand trial before Caesar.

✞ What does "press on" mean to you?

✞ Do you feel you can press on when your days are so filled with health concerns? If so, how? If not, why not?

✞ What is your goal in life: to get through each day, to do the good things God has planned for me, to adjust my attitude to fit my circumstances, to accept each moment as it comes, to develop lasting relationships? Explain.

JOURNAL: ISA. 58 WHAT DOES GOD'S FAST LOOK LIKE? HOW CAN YOU MEET THESE REQUIREMENTS? DO YOU?

Heavenly Promises #7

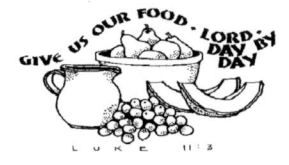

⁸For physical training is of some value, but godliness has value for all things, holding promise for both the present life and the life to come. ⁹ This is a trustworthy saying that deserves full acceptance. (1 Tim. 4:8-9)

✤ What physical activities have you had to give up due to your illness? How does this make you feel?

✤ Easton's Illustrated (Biblical) Dictionary states that godliness "supposes knowledge, veneration, affection, dependence, submission, gratitude, and obedience." What does "godliness" look like to you?

✤ There is a saying, "Cleanliness is next to godliness!" After reflecting on the meaning of godliness, what do you think about this statement? Rewrite or rephrase this declaration.

✤ Do you agree with Paul that godliness is for both the present and the future? How can that be?

JOURNAL: 1 TIM. 6 DOES YOUR HEALTH AFFECT YOUR FINANCES? WHEN DOES MONEY GET IN THE WAY OF GODLINESS? EXPLAIN.

Paul: Heavenly Minded #8

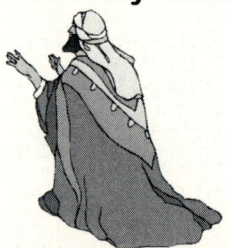

For our struggle is not against flesh and blood, but against the rulers, against the authorities, against the powers of this dark world and against the spiritual forces of evil in the heavenly realms. (Eph. 6:12)

Paul's ocean voyage to Rome was eventful. The ship encountered a vicious storm that eventually broke it apart. All through the storm, Paul encouraged the men that not one soul would be lost because God had assured Paul he would reach Rome and stand trial before Caesar. (Acts 27)

☦ Who or what are the "spiritual forces of evil"? Where do they rule? What can you do about them?

☦ Paul recognized that his fiercest battles were not physical but spiritual. What spiritual issues are you fighting: pride, fear, greed, unforgiveness, lust, gluttony, etc.?

☦ How do you battle spiritual concerns when you must also contend with physical circumstances?

JOURNAL: PS. 86 DOES THIS PSALM ENCOURAGE YOU IN YOUR STRUGGLE WITH ILLNESS? EXPLAIN.

Heavenly Promises #8

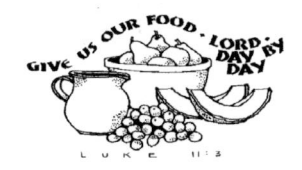

The Lord will rescue me from every evil attack and will bring me safely to his heavenly kingdom. To him be glory for ever and ever. Amen. (2 Tim. 4:18)

✞ Do you see your illness as an evil attack? Explain.

✞ When has God rescued you recently? How?

✞ 2 Chron. 20:17, in part states, **You will not have to fight this battle... stand firm and see the deliverance the Lord will give you... Do not be afraid; do not be discouraged...** Each day can be a battle when dealing with chronic illness. What battle will you ask the Lord to fight for you today?

✞ What does your "stand firm" look like when dealing with life-altering, physical pain?

✞ How do you fight the discouragement that often comes with continual pain?

JOURNAL: ISA. 40:25-31 IN WHOM DOES YOUR STRENGTH LIE? HOW CAN YOU ACCESS THIS POWER?

Paul: Heavenly Minded #9

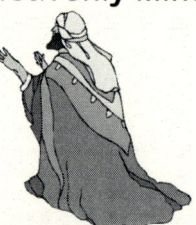

Jesus said: *¹⁷And these signs will accompany those who believe: In my name they will drive out demons; they will speak in new tongues; ¹⁸ they will pick up snakes with their hands; and when they drink deadly poison, it will not hurt them at all; they will place their hands on sick people, and they will get well.* (Mark 16:17-18)

Shipwrecked on Malta, Paul gathered wood for a fire, and was bitten by a deadly viper. Instead of swelling up and dying, he shook off the snake with no ill effects. (Acts 28)

☦ Jesus' words do not encourage us to pick up snakes or drink poison. The event on Malta puts His words in perspective. Certainly, bad things happen to believers. Why is this?

☦ When have you experienced a medical condition that you could "shake off"? If never, then how do you cope?

☦ It is not the amount of faith we have that permits healing. Healing is God's choice. What spiritual or emotional healing have you experienced? Is it enough?

JOURNAL: JOHN 16:22-33 IS THERE JOY IN PAIN? EXPLAIN.

Heavenly Promises #9

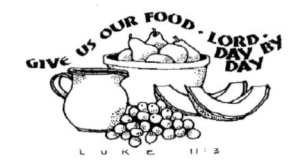

Therefore, holy brothers, who share in the heavenly calling, fix your thoughts on Jesus, the apostle and high priest whom we confess. (Heb. 3:1)

☫ What meaning does "heavenly calling" have for you?

☫ The verse before Heb. 3:1 is Heb. 2:18: ***Because he*** [Jesus] ***himself suffered when he was tempted, he is able to help those who are being tempted.*** What temptations do you think Jesus endured?

☫ What types of temptations do you suffer? How do you overcome these temptations? Are you successful?

☫ How can Jesus "help those who are being tempted"? How can He help you?

☫ When does fixing your thoughts on Jesus help?

JOURNAL: PS. 141 WHEN TEMPTATION HOUNDS YOU, HOW DOES GOD HELP YOU OVERCOME THE IMPULSE? DO YOU ACCEPT GOD'S HELP OR IGNORE IT?

Paul: Heavenly Minded #10

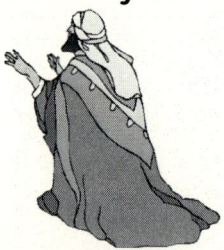

¹²I know what it is to be in need, and I know what it is to have plenty. I have learned the secret of being content in any and every situation, whether well fed or hungry, whether living in plenty or in want. ¹³ I can do everything through him who gives me strength. (Phil. 4:12-13)

In Rome, while chained to guards day and night, Paul received visitors and continually preached the truth of Jesus Christ. Though soldiers were frequently rotated, many of Caesar's household became saved. (Phil. 4:22)

✞ Which situations listed by Paul have you personally experienced? How did you feel during those times?

✞ How well do you respond to being hungry or deprived? Are you encouraged by your response? If not, what can you do to modify your reaction to hardships?

✞ Where can you acquire skills to make it through difficult circumstances and challenging relationships?

JOURNAL: JOHN 6:35-40 HOW EFFECTIVELY DOES JESUS SATISFY YOUR HUNGER, NEEDS, AND WANTS?

Heavenly Promises #10

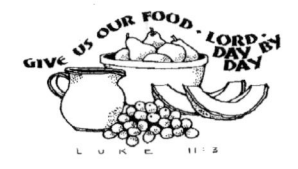

Instead, they [martyrs] *were longing for a better country--a heavenly one. Therefore God is not ashamed to be called their God, for he has prepared a city for them.* (Heb. 11:16)

✞ What physical or spiritual occurrence are you longing for right now? Explain why.

✞ Have you ever been ashamed to declare that you are a Christian? When and why? If not, how have you stood against the skepticism found in today's culture?

✞ Death is something that every living thing experiences. Do you ever think of dying? What are your thoughts? If you are not concerned, why not?

✞ Describe the new city of God waiting for you when you die.

JOURNAL: 1 PETER 3:8-17 WHAT ADVICE DO THESE VERSES GIVE YOU THAT APPLIES TO YOUR LIFE RIGHT NOW? WHAT MUST YOU DO? HOW CAN YOUR FEAR INTERFERE?

LEADER'S GUIDE

Through my own experiences as leader of chronic pain support groups, I have learned that God chooses who will be in my Bible studies. Members become as important to me as they do to each other. I may be the facilitator and teacher, but I am also called upon to be a confidant, a port in the storm, a hand holder, a shoulder to cry on, and a boo-boo kisser. These precious saints arouse compassion, require empathy, erase pity, and demand validation as they inspire, support, motivate, and stretch me as well as each other. God brings us together because we need one another.

Now you have heard God's voice calling you to minister, and you are willing to take on a most challenging good work. You have seized the opportunity to facilitate a group of physically hurting people, to teach them how to apply God's words to their lives, to encourage them to break out of their confining lives of pain, to offer them a forum in which they may be heard and not judged, and to build them into a supportive community through laughter, tears, tolerance, and shared experiences.

Before you begin, recognize that participants must expend a great amount of energy just to get to the meetings, that special accommodations may be necessary, that physical comfort is crucial, that a routine needs to be set in place at once, and that trust must be established quickly.

This Bible study may be unlike any you have ever attempted. Lessons are short, questions are intense, and application of Scripture is essential. Provide "thinking time" for each person to consider the question carefully. Guide them toward self-application and not using other people's experiences. Finally, expect each person to learn the Scripture Memory verse, since you will spend weeks learning each verse piece by piece. Encourage your group to embrace the verse(s) in their daily struggle with frustrating, painful situations.

Suggested Framework:

- meet weekly, it's easier to establish a routine for participants, especially scheduling dr. appointments
- require no written homework but suggest that questions need to be read and thought about before coming to group
- time of day is critical: too early and members can't get out of bed, too late and the day has worn them out
- length of focused time no longer than ninety minutes:
   - ✓ 30 minutes for sharing, building community, revealing answered prayers and reciting last week's memory verse (allows for tardiness)
   - ✓ 30 minutes for study time using the book
   - ✓ 30 minutes for praises, prayer requests, and new Scripture verse, or section, to memorize

Commitment expected from members:

Having expectations encourages member efforts to comply. Create an atmosphere where each person is important to the group's effectiveness. This study is not a drop-in event but a significant part of each member's life.

- be on time (recognize this will not always happen)
- attend each week
- pray for and with each other
- apply Scripture to daily challenges
- attempt to learn the weekly Scripture memory verse

Rules for sharing:

- don't try to fix anyone
- share only what works for you
- don't make suggestions like, "Have you tried…"
- everything shared in the group stays in the group
- suggestions for treatments, medications, holistic methods, etc. can be shared after the meeting

Pitfalls to watch out for:

- pity-parties, blaming others, and/or complaining
- prayer requests for other people and not for self
- one person's drama consuming all of group time
- non-attendance judged or criticized
- Bible study turns into counseling sessions

Leader preparation:

The Old Testament tells the story of God refining His chosen people, the Israelites, in preparation for the arrival of the Messiah, Jesus Christ, who would take upon Himself the sins of humanity. The Salvation we gain through Christ allows mankind to once again have fellowship with Holy God. Though God chose a nation, it is the personal relationship He had with individuals that reveals His intention to have a personal relationship with each of us. Thus, intimacy with Christ, His one-on-one availability, is stressed throughout all four chapters of this book.

Therefore, though we can learn from any character in the Bible, I chose to focus on these four men. From Joseph we learn that our circumstances do not have to determine our faith. From Moses we learn that faint hearts can become emboldened through praise. From Nehemiah we learn to pray first then act, and that one needs to bless God and not curse one's infirmities. Lastly, we learn from Paul to act on

God's promises and not be defeated by the worries of the world.

There are advantages to reading or rereading each man's complete story, but it is not necessary. If you are so inclined, though, you can find Joseph in chapters 37-50 in the book of Genesis, Moses in the book of Exodus, Nehemiah in the book of Nehemiah, and Paul, first called Saul, in Acts 8:1-3, 9:1-32, and in Acts chapters 13-28.

Memorizing Scripture:

Memorizing Scripture and applying it to our daily lives cannot be stressed enough. It is surprising how often pieces of Scripture floating in one's brain can make all the difference in dealing with a painful or traumatic situation. Encourage your members during the first 30 minutes of community building to share how they applied the memory verse during the last week.

Memorizing Scripture is hard for most everyone; but for those in pain, it is a mountain they think they cannot climb. Therefore, I have developed several helpful techniques that are useful for various styles of learning. Be sure to use the same Bible version throughout when memorizing.

> #1: Read together the entire memory verse from the Bible. Copy it using 3X5 cards—you say the verse in small phrases: "Matt. 6:33"—pause—"But seek first his kingdom"—pause then repeat "But seek first his kingdom"—pause—"and his righteousness"—pause and repeat etc. At the end repeat the address, "Matt. 6:33" Some members will want to copy the verse while you speak it and others will copy straight from the Bible. Read cards together when everyone is finished. Emphasize accuracy in this step.

#2: Discuss the meaning of the verse by reading it in the context from which it came, i.e. What does "all things" mean?

#3: Discuss where members can tape the 3X5 card so that they will see it frequently, i.e. refrigerator, car, etc.

#4: Encourage them to personalize the verse, i.e. "I will seek first God's kingdom and His righteousness."

#5: Choose a small phrase to learn each week. For example, in Phil. 4:6 start them with the phrase, "Do not be anxious about anything" Ask them to apply that phrase this week so that they may share next week.

#6: As each week progresses, you will add to the Scripture, one phrase at a time, i.e. to "Do not be anxious about anything" you will add, "but in everything."

#7: Point out punctuation and phrases, i.e. in Phil. 4:6 there are four commas and five phrases which means that it will take at least five weeks for the group to complete memorizing this Scripture.

#8: Call attention to repetition of words or similar phrases, i.e. in Ps. 27:1 both sentences start with, "The Lord." The end of each sentence is similar, "whom shall I..." and "of whom shall I..."

#9: Use gimmicks such as drawing pictures for words, either mental or on paper, i.e. "my light" engenders an image of a light bulb, "stronghold" brings to mind a fortress. One young lady declared the perfect image for "my salvation" was chocolate. None of us forgot this verse!

You will surprise yourself by adding even more techniques to this list as your group evolves.

CHAPTER ONE--LEADER'S GUIDE

Victimized by Circumstances or Rejuvenated by Faith

Chapter Emphasis:
- Joseph was unable to control his circumstances, yet his choice of faith in God's laws allowed him to be effective no matter what his situation.
- Participants may not be able to control their chronic illness, but they are able to choose to declare God's promises as they respond to their daily challenges.

Scripture Memory Verse(s): (Feel free to choose other verses to meet your own group's needs)
- Matt. 6:33 (approx. 4 weeks)
- Phil. 4:6 (approx. 5-6 weeks)

Leader's Background Reading for Each Lesson:
- Joseph #1: Gen. 37:1-11
- Joseph #2: Gen. 37:12-35
- Joseph #3: Gen. 39:1-6
- Joseph #4: Gen. 39:6-18
- Joseph #5: Gen. 39:19-23
- Joseph #6: Gen. 40:1-23
- Joseph #7: Gen. 41:1-32
- Joseph #8: Gen. 41:33-57
- Joseph #9: Gen. 42 & 43
- Joseph #10: Gen. 44 & 45

CHAPTER TWO--LEADER'S GUIDE

Make a Loud Noise or Sing a New Song

Chapter Emphasis:

- Moses chose to limit his life to what he could see and understand. In spite of this, God called him to an enormous task beyond his capabilities. Moses started out with excuses but ended choosing a new attitude.

- Participants may see themselves only in terms of their illness. This perspective makes their lives very small. Familiarity with God's truths allows them the choice to "change their tune."

Scripture Memory Verse(s):

- 2 Cor. 4:16-18 (approx. 10 weeks)

Leader's Background Reading for Each Lesson:

- Moses #1: Ex. 2 & 3:1-12
- Moses #2: Ex. 3:13-22
- Moses #3: Ex. 4:1-12
- Moses #4: Ex. 4:13-31
- Moses #5: Ex. 5
- Moses #6: Ex. 6 & 7:1-6 (Chap. 7-12 are the plagues)
- Moses #7: Ex. 13-14
- Moses #8: Ex. 15
- Moses #9: Deut. 31:15-29
- Moses #10: Deut. 32:1-47

CHAPTER THREE--LEADER'S GUIDE

Cursed by Enemies or Blessed by God

Chapter Emphasis:

- Nehemiah was a man of purpose who prayed before he took action. His enemies were relentless, but his choices allowed him to complete a seemingly impossible task.
- Chronic illness oftentimes may seem to be a curse. By focusing on the ability to adjust their attitudes, participants may be able to focus on the blessings in their lives instead of on their difficulties.

Scripture Memory Verse(s):

- 2 Chron. 20:17 (approx. 10 weeks)

Leader's Background Reading for Each Lesson:

- Nehemiah #1: Neh. 1
- Nehemiah #2: Neh. 2:1-10
- Nehemiah #3: Neh. 2:11-17
- Nehemiah #4: Neh. 2:18-20
- Nehemiah #5: Neh. 4:1-6
- Nehemiah #6: Neh. 4:7-10
- Nehemiah #7: Neh. 4:11-22
- Nehemiah #8: Neh. 6:1-14
- Nehemiah #9: Neh. 6:15-19
- Nehemiah #10: Neh. 13:6-22

CHAPTER FOUR--LEADER'S GUIDE

Worldly Cares or Heavenly Promises

Chapter Emphasis:

- Paul's suffering was undiminished as he spread the news of to the Gentile world. He who could do miraculous healing of others could not be healed himself. God had a higher purpose for Paul's suffering. Paul chose to accept, and not fight, his weaknesses so that God's power could be revealed.

- Participants can choose to live beyond the limitations of their physical illness and to discover how God's promises are applicable to their lives.

Scripture Memory Verse(s):

- Prov. 3:5-6 (approx. 4 weeks)
- Heb. 12:1b (approx. 6 weeks)

Leader's Background Reading for Each Lesson:
- Paul #1: Acts 9
- Paul #2: Acts 14:8-20
- Paul #3: 2Cor. 11:22-30, 12:7-10
- Paul #4: Acts 16:16-24
- Paul #5: Acts 16: 25-40
- Paul #6: Acts 21:30-22:22
- Paul #7: Acts 22:22-29, 25:1-12, 26:32
- Paul #8: Acts 27
- Paul #9: Acts 28:1-10
- Paul #10: Acts 28:11-30

SERIES: GOD'S Rx FOR CHRONIC PAIN

Book One — *THE SILVER BULLET: GOD'S Rx FOR CHRONIC PAIN*

Chapter 1: God Declares Jesus Is His Son
Chapter 2: God Identifies Jesus With Many Names
Chapter 3: God Provides Jesus As Our Savior
Chapter 4: God Affirms That Jesus Is The Way To Him

Book Two — *CHOICES: MANAGING CHRONIC PAIN*

Chapter 1: Victimized By Circumstances Or Rejuvenated By Faith
Chapter 2: Make A Loud Noise Or Sing A New Song
Chapter 3: Curse Your Enemies Or Bless Your God
Chapter 4: Worldly Cares Or Heavenly Promises

BOOKS TO COME

Book Three — *THE VINEYARD: GROWING THROUGH CHRONIC PAIN*

Chapter 1: The Gardener
Chapter 2: The True Vine
Chapter 3: The Fruit
Chapter 4: The Pruning

Book Four — *MOUNTAIN CLIMBING: POSSIBILITIES DESPITE CHRONIC PAIN*

Chapter 1: Jesus, Guide To Impossible Mountain Climbing
Chapter 2: Jesus, Escort Through Suffering
Chapter 3: Jesus, Encouragement Through Anxiety
Chapter 4: Jesus, Restoration To Climbers